The HIIT Advantage

High-Intensity Workouts for Women

Irene Lewis-McCormick

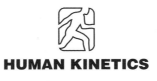

HUMAN KINETICS

Library of Congress Cataloging-in-Publication Data

Lewis-McCormick, Irene, 1967-
    The HIIT advantage : high-intensity workouts for women / Irene Lewis-McCormick.
        pages cm
    Includes bibliographical references and index.
    1. Reducing exercises. 2. Exercise for women. 3. Physical fitness. 4. Weight training. I. Title.
    RA781.6.L49 2016

    613.7'1082--dc23

                                                        2015018430

ISBN: 978-1-4925-0306-4 (print)

Acquisitions Editor: Michelle Maloney; **Developmental Editor:** Laura Pulliam; **Managing Editor:** Nicole O'Dell; **Copyeditor:** Patsy Fortney; **Indexer:** Bobbi Swanson; **Senior Graphic Designer:** Fred Starbird; **Cover Designer:** Keith Blomberg; **Photographs (cover and interior):** Neil Bernstein; **Video Producer:** Doug Fink; **Visual Production Coordinator:** Joyce Brumfield; **Photo Production Manager:** Jason Allen; **Art Manager:** Kelly Hendren; **Associate Art Manager:** Alan L. Wilborn; **Illustrations:** © Human Kinetics; **Printer:** Sheridan Books

We thank Fitness World North in Ankeny, Iowa, for assistance in providing the location for the photo shoot for this book.
Human Kinetics books are available at special discounts for bulk purchase. Special editions or book excerpts can also be created to specification. For details, contact the Special Sales Manager at Human Kinetics.

The video contents of this product are licensed for private home use and traditional, face-to-face classroom instruction only. For public performance licensing, please contact a sales representative at www.HumanKinetics.com/SalesRepresentatives.

Printed in the United States of America   10 9 8 7 6 5 4 3 2 1

The paper in this book is certified under a sustainable forestry program.

11-18-15   OCLC

Human Kinetics
Website: www.HumanKinetics.com

United States: Human Kinetics
P.O. Box 5076
Champaign, IL 61825-5076
800-747-4457
e-mail: humank@hkusa.com

Canada: Human Kinetics
475 Devonshire Road Unit 100
Windsor, ON N8Y 2L5
800-465-7301 (in Canada only)
e-mail: info@hkcanada.com

Europe: Human Kinetics
107 Bradford Road
Stanningley
Leeds LS28 6AT, United Kingdom
+44 (0) 113 255 5665
e-mail: hk@hkeurope.com

Australia: Human Kinetics
57A Price Avenue
Lower Mitcham, South Australia 5062
08 8372 0999
e-mail: info@hkaustralia.com

New Zealand: Human Kinetics
P.O. Box 80
Mitcham Shopping Centre, South Australia 5062
0800 222 062
e-mail: info@hknewzealand.com

E6397

This book is dedicated to the fitness professionals
who commit themselves daily to long hours
as they motivate, educate, and inspire others.

CONTENTS

PART I

HIGH-INTENSITY INTERVAL TRAINING, HIGH-INTENSITY RESULTS

CHAPTER **1**   Understanding HIIT . . . .

Become familiar with how high-intensity interval training differs from other forms of exercise, and why HIIT works to achieve maximum results in minimal time.

CHAPTER **2**   Role of Recovery . . . .

Explore the types of post-exercise recovery and their benefits in improving performance and decreasing injury risk.

CHAPTER **3**   Popular HIIT Protocols . . . .

Learn the differences among HIIT protocols, when to use them, and how to determine which are best to meet your unique needs.

CHAPTER **4**   Incorporating Tools and Toys . . . .

Add variety and challenge to your HIIT workouts with fun and portable fitness equipment.

PART II

HIGH-INTENSITY INTERVAL EXERCISES

CHAPTER **5**   Lower-Body Exercises . . . .

Identify effective exercises that are critical for balance, support, and stability, and that work major muscles to burn calories and increase lean muscle mass.

PART **III**

HIGH-INTENSITY INTERVAL WORKOUTS

VIDEO CONTENTS

LOWER-BODY EXERCISES

ACCESSING THE ONLINE VIDEO

This book includes access to online video that includes 24 clips demonstrating dynamic exercises presented in the book and one full 30-minute HIIT workout. Throughout the book, exercises marked with this play button icon ⏵ indicate where the content is enhanced by online video clips.

Take the following steps to access the video. If you need help at any point in the process, you can contact us by clicking on the Technical Support link under Customer Service on the right side of the screen.

1. Visit www.HumanKinetics.com/TheHIITAdvantage.
2. Click on the **View online video link** next to the book cover.
3. You will be directed to the screen shown in figure 1. Click the **Sign In link** on the left or top of the page. If you do not have an account with Human Kinetics, you will be prompted to create one.

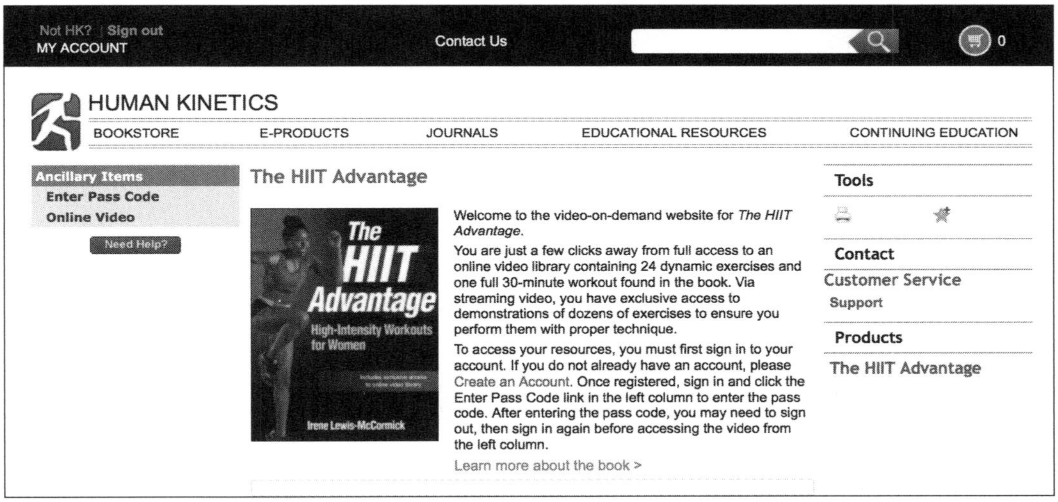

Figure 1

4. If the online video does not appear in the list on the left of the page, click the **Enter Pass Code** option in that list. Enter the pass code exactly as it is printed here, including all hyphens. Click the **Submit** button to unlock the online video. After you have entered this pass code the first time, you will never have to enter it again. For future visits, all you need to do is sign in to the book's website and follow the link that appears in the left menu.

Pass code for online video: LEWISMCCOR-4T3P-OV

5. Once you have signed into the site and entered the pass code, select **Online Video** from the list on the left side of the screen. You'll then see an Online Video page with information about the video, as shown in the screenshot in figure 2. You can go straight to the accompanying videos for each topic by clicking on the blue links at the bottom of the page.

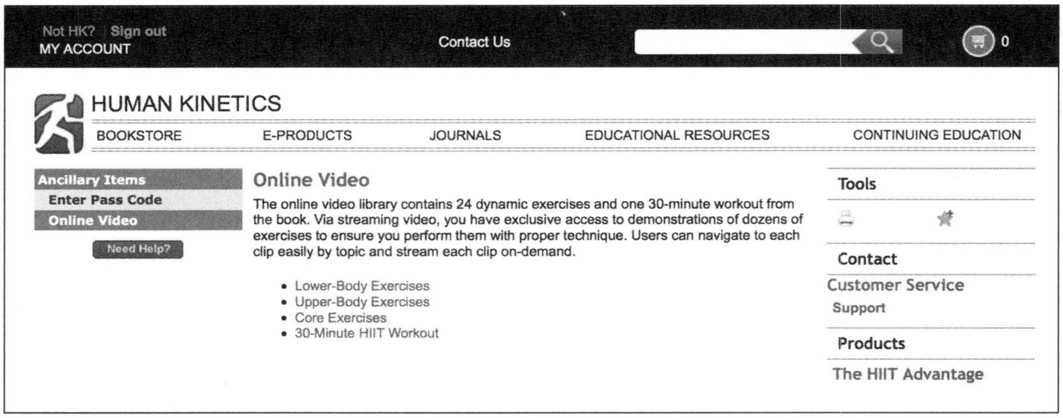

Figure 2

6. You are now able to view video for the topic you selected on the previous screen, as well as others that accompany this product. Across the top of this page, you will see a set of buttons that correspond to the topics in the text that have accompanying video:

Lower-Body Exercises

Upper-Body Exercises

Core Exercises

30-Minute HIIT Workout

Once you click on a topic, a player will appear. In the player, the clips for that topic will appear vertically along the right side. Select the video you would like to watch and view it in the main player window. You can use the buttons at the bottom of the main player window to view the video full screen, to turn captioning on and off, and to pause, fast-forward, or reverse the clip.

PREFACE

As high-intensity interval training (HIIT) programs have proliferated in the fitness industry, an obvious need has developed for a complete application-based text with an explanation of what HIIT is and how it can be used to enhance training. Not nearly enough information exists in a single source regarding how to use HIIT for everyday fitness. This book contains information about taking a decisive approach to HIIT and manipulating the energy systems with purposeful exercises that include built-in progressions and regressions that are quick, effective, and can bring about major changes. Exercise selections focus on major calorie burning, increased lean muscle, and fat loss for women at any fitness level.

Most articles and studies that examine HIIT are geared toward researchers, coaches, and fitness professionals; they address the physiology of HIIT, how it is used for elite athletes, and often its physical benefits. Additionally, most articles focus mainly on the Tabata approach, but HIIT is much more than just going super hard. Moreover, it is more than just a trend or fad. HIIT is a specific system based on scientific research and an outgrowth of increased knowledge in the areas of functional, continuous interval training using regular ratios of training to recovery. Even though this book is detailed enough to assist and guide a highly skilled trainer or coach, it is designed to be a handbook for women who may be less familiar with HIIT, or have minimal experience using HIIT protocols. Although written for women, this book is for anyone of any fitness level who want to use HIIT to achieve consistent results and amazing benefits. HIIT is the next logical step in the future of exercise, weight loss, increased stamina, and strength and performance enhancement for fitness enthusiasts of all ages and fitness levels.

Making a complex topic like HIIT seem simple and easy to follow or implement is challenging, yet that is the intention of this book. It is the first complete collection of HIIT protocols for female fitness professionals and female fitness consumers alike. Anyone who wants to enhance an exercise routine, boost overall health, and increase performance-based fitness can use this book. The selected HIIT protocols are explained fully, and intensity strategies are provided based on your fitness level and personal goals. These workouts can be used to increase power, endurance, and strength, and they highlight the importance of recovery and its role in performance enhancement and injury prevention. To simplify this complex topic, this book offers 16 easy-to-follow workouts that are safe and effective.

The initial chapters explain HIIT and continuous interval training protocols, describe the rationale behind them, and address the role and importance of recovery. We examine the Tabata intervals known as max, mixed, and timed, as well as the hard, harder, hardest format, an ascending time-based protocol that increases movement intensity while decreasing duration. Chapter 4 highlights portable equipment that can be used during HIIT workouts, including dumbbells and resistance tubing. Subsequent chapters highlight the exercises and combinations of exercises that comprise the HIIT workouts by body region: lower body, upper body, and core. Chapter 8 provides a menu of options for using the suggested routines.

Photographs and streaming video enhance the experience of learning HIIT by bringing the exercises to life. The exercises that have accompanying video are

listed in the video contents and are also marked with this symbol in the text:
All the exercises are described fully in easy-to-follow 20-, 30-, and 45-minute
HIIT routines, depending on how much time you have to exercise. There are even 30
max interval options, single-movement exercises that you can do any day of the week
in 4-minute increments; these are particularly helpful when you are time-pressed or
just want to add a little extra boost to your daily routine. The most important aspect
of this book is that it is for the exerciser—the person who wants to apply science and
research to a fitness program without having to wade through all the scientific jargon.

The HIIT Advantage is a one-stop-shopping experience that provides a complete,
effective, and results-based training program for women of all fitness levels. Readers
will be coached to make the exercises work by using progressions, regressions, and
even modifications when necessary. On-ramps and off-ramps to increase or decrease
intensity are incorporated into every movement pattern in each exercise routine, so
that a customized workout that meets your current skill set and fitness level can be
achieved.

Stop spinning your wheels using tired, ineffective workouts that promote overuse,
fatigue, and do not create overload. Instead, use these training techniques to include
intensity and variety to consistently challenge your body each and every workout. Use
the workouts in this book to see significant improvements in performance including
increased fat loss, improved aerobic stamina, enhanced anaerobic capacity, and greater
strength and power. This book will serve as an integral part of your fitness training,
teaching exercises you can use now and as an ongoing resource after. Start working
smarter and harder, in less time, for better results. *The HIIT Advantage* focuses on
protocols for better physical performance and appearance with exercise designed
with specific purpose for predictable outcomes. Work harder and smarter and get
results in less time, because more is not better; *better is better.*

ACKNOWLEDGMENTS

I would like to take this opportunity to thank some wonderful people who have influenced and inspired me over the course of my 30-plus-year career as a fitness professional. There is no way I could include every person, because there are too many, but with respect to high-intensity interval training and the publication of this book in particular, I would specifically like to thank Bruce and Mindy Mylrea of the brilliant and forward-thinking total-wellness program known as Tabata Bootcamp. They were the first in the fitness industry to put HIIT into everyday workouts for real people in a manageable and effective format. Mindy is a constant inspiration to me and taught me what I needed to know to write this book. She continues to partner with her husband, Bruce, in encouraging others to change their lives through nutrition and small- and large-group HIIT programs across the globe.

I would also like to acknowledge the excellent people at RYKA, especially Todd Murray and Rachel Zakoura, who generously donated the shoes made just for women that all the beautiful models wore in our extensive photo sessions.

I'd like to thank my supervisor and friend, Nancy Shaw, of the City of Ames Parks & Recreation. I appreciate her support, encouragement, and trust in my program design and coaching skills and her constant accommodation of my very demanding schedule.

Thanks to the people at Human Kinetics, specifically Laura Pulliam for her editing expertise and Michelle Maloney for guiding me through the entire process. And last I'd like to thank my loving and supportive husband, Sean, and my two beautiful and talented daughters, Madeleine and Delaney, who are a constant source of support, inspiration, and encouragement to me so I can do what I love.

PART

HIGH-INTENSITY INTERVAL TRAINING, HIGH-INTENSITY RESULTS

UNDERSTANDING HIIT

HIIT stands for *high-intensity interval training,* also known as a burst and recovery cycle. In standard HIIT, very high-intensity anaerobic eruptions of movement are paired with low-effort, rest intervals. This type of exercise offers powerful intensity to improve cardiorespiratory and muscular fitness, but it doesn't stop there. HIIT rewards the body in many ways, including boosting athletic performance, improving overall health, and providing many of the other weight loss and wellness benefits seen with traditional steady-state endurance training. HIIT protocols have also been shown to increase glucose metabolism, an important component in energy use as well as fat burning.

Sound too good to be true? It's not, really, because the trade-off is that HIIT requires maximal effort—you will be performing really hard work for short bursts of time with minimal rest between. You will definitely earn every rest period you get. HIIT sessions can vary in length from 4 to 45 minutes, and although this may seem out of reach for some, it isn't because high-intensity interval training can be performed in so many ways. It can be customized to meet you at your current fitness level and help you achieve the results you are looking for.

This book demonstrates the variety of HIIT options, including several ways to build up to working harder and harder over time in each burst and recovery cycle. You can use both body-weight and equipment in the exercises, as well as a variety of interval timing protocols. The exercises and workouts in this book include safe and effective movements in a format that is right for you regardless of your level of fitness.

HISTORY OF HIIT

Although HIIT is very popular today, it is not exactly a new concept. It is most commonly called HIIT, but it has also been referred to as HIIE (high-intensity intermittent exercise), as well as SIT (sprint interval training), particularly in track and field. As early as 1912, the Finnish Olympic runner Hannes Kolehmainen was using HIIT protocols in his pursuit of Olympic Gold. In 1970, Peter Coe, inspired by the sprint training performed by professor Woldemar Gerschler of Germany and Per-Olof Åstrand of Sweden, used a SIT regimen in the training of his son Sebastian Coe; it consisted of repeated 200-meter runs with 30 seconds of rest between them. Sebastian Coe went on to achieve great success as an Olympic athlete, making and breaking several records in middle-distance events including the 800- and 1,500-meter runs.

In the 1930s, a protocol was developed called fartlek training; *fartlek* is Swedish for "speed play." The fartlek method involves continuous, steady-state, and discontinuous interval training, which allows the athlete to run at various intensities at personally chosen distances. The Gibala regimen, also known as the Little method, was created by professor Martin Gibala and Jonathan Little; it consists of a 3-minute warm-up followed by 60 seconds of intense exercise (at 90 percent of $\dot{V}O_2$max) followed by 75 seconds of rest, which is repeated for 8 to 12 cycles.

In 1996 the most popular version of HIIT, called Tabata, was researched and developed by professor Izumi Tabata. This training was initially used with Olympic speedskaters and performed on a stationary cycle. In his research, Tabata had athletes perform 20 seconds of ultra-high-intensity cycling (at 170 percent of $\dot{V}O_2$max) for 20 seconds followed by 10 seconds of rest. This was repeated for 4 minutes, so the athletes performed 8 rounds (Tabata, et al, 1996). Many fitness professionals have adapted this protocol to their athletes' and clients' training repertoires with enormous success, and Tabata has become one of the most popular HIIT formats to date. The major advantage of Tabata protocols comes from the high-intensity burst effective at improving both the aerobic and the anaerobic capacities, which provides performance results in short time frames for a wide range of athletic endeavors.

WHY HIIT?

As mentioned, HIIT can offer amazing health and fitness benefits using workouts that are shorter and performed less often than aerobic activities, in which improvements come with a greater volume of training, meaning more time running, swimming, cycling, or using an aerobic machine such as a treadmill. The greatest appeal of HIIT is its time-saving attributes, but the benefits go much further to include a cumulative, broad range of physiological gains in both health and performance.

HIIT Versus Discontinuous Interval Training

For several years, research has consistently shown that interval training increases overall levels of fitness and burns more calories over a short period of time as compared with steady-state aerobic exercise. In the past, the traditional approach to interval training typically consisted of cardio workouts that alternated steady-state exercise with higher workloads (intervals) for short periods and provided positive recovery periods in a variety of time frames. For example, in the traditional interval approach, you determine the length and speed of each high-intensity interval based on how you feel that day. After warming up, you might increase the intensity for 30 seconds and then resume your normal aerobic pace. The next burst of more intense activity may last 2 to 3 minutes. The intensity and how often you change or add an interval and for how long are largely determined by you.

This personally established approach to interval training is referred to as discontinuous interval training because, unless otherwise specified, the approach to each interval and recovery period is neither systematic nor controlled. Such an approach to interval training is useful, because it offers exercisers the flexibility to intersperse harder bouts of discontinuous loads of high-intensity movements with lower-intensity recovery periods and helps improve anaerobic as well as aerobic capacity, but in much longer training sessions with much lower microbursts of intensity. However, unlike HIIT, traditional discontinuous interval training does not consist of precise, specific time frames in which to perform the higher-intensity workloads and is not necessarily systematic.

In the HIIT protocols presented in this book, the interval ratios are clearly prescribed, detailed, and specific. Additionally, the concept of negative recovery is a major difference between the more random approach of discontinuous interval training and HIIT. Because of the negative aspect of recovery in precise ratios, HIIT is harder and can yield greater training results.

HIIT Versus Steady-State Training

Research has demonstrated the effectiveness of HIIT protocols by contrasting them with steady-state endurance, or aerobic, exercise. To appreciate the power of HIIT, it's important to understand the difference between steady-state, aerobic endurance activities and high-intensity exercise.

Steady-state aerobic activity, or endurance exercise, is simply a form of cardio exercise paced at a continuous, steady rate. This can be defined as exercise performed continuously, such as walking or running for at least 20 minutes at a pace at which oxygen supply meets oxygen demand; the heart rate stays at a constant pace and you do not become breathless. During a HIIT protocol, on the other hand, you vary your energy output and become breathless, or close to it, for short periods of time. $\dot{V}O_2$max is considered the body's upper limit for consuming and distributing oxygen for the purpose of energy production and is considered a good predictor of exercise performance. $\dot{V}O_2$max is also considered the gold standard for determining peak power output, or the maximal physical work capacity a person is capable of. For most healthy people, the $\dot{V}O_2$max during a steady-state workout is somewhere between 50 and 70 percent. The rate of oxygen consumption increases as the level of intensity increases—for example, from rest to easy, from easy to difficult, and from difficult to maximal effort.

Additionally, the cardiovascular system adapts to aerobic stressors by increasing in functional capacity. The application of a stressor in exercise science terminology is referred to as overload. When a system of the body (e.g., the cardiovascular system) is overloaded through aerobic activity, it responds by becoming stronger, more resilient, and better able to handle the stress of greater activity and at more intense levels. Aerobic overload results in a stronger heart muscle, improved lung capacity, and better overall cardiorespiratory performance. These parameters are measured by heart rate, stroke volume, and the contractility (the ability to contract with force) of the heart muscle. These factors also assist in blood flow, which allows the oxygen supply to meet the oxygen and energy demands of the working muscles during aerobic activities.

However, there are more than just heart health rewards to be gained from aerobic exercise. The list of benefits is actually quite long. They include increased contraction of skeletal muscles, which also boosts blood flow, making venous blood return to the heart more efficient. This quicker return of blood to the heart increases how quickly blood can refill in the ventricles (the chambers of the heart), which results in an increased preload. This elevated preload adds to the heart's ability to expel blood quickly, which in turn contributes significantly to enhanced aerobic performance. The following physiological markers are just a few more of the many benefits of aerobic activity:

• Increased size of heart muscle (stronger heart)
• Increased stroke volume (more blood flows out with each heartbeat)

- Increased rate of oxidized enzyme efficiency (creates ATP energy with greater efficiency)
- Increased rate and efficiency of oxygen and fuel getting into muscle
- Greater endurance of slow-twitch muscle fibers (Type I, slower to fatigue)
- Increased reliance on fat as an energy source
- Increased number of mitochondria (energy factory of a muscle cell)
- Better ability to dispose of waste products created in the muscles during exercise (onset of blood lactate accumulation, or OBLA)

But even with all this evidence demonstrating the positive effects of aerobic activities, much of the newer research is demonstrating that HIIT protocols provide the same health and performance benefits, and more. A study performed by Helgerud and colleagues (2007) showed that HIIT was significantly more effective in improving maximal oxygen uptake ($\dot{V}O_2$max) and stroke volume (the amount of blood that pumps out of the left ventricle each time the heart beats) than steady-state aerobic activity.

Another study examined participants who performed a HIIT walking workout (walking on a treadmill at 80 to 90 percent of $\dot{V}O_2$max) 3 times a week for 10 weeks. These participants were compared with a control group who performed an aerobic walking program at 50 to 60 percent of $\dot{V}O_2$max. The HIIT group had a 12 percent increase in the size of the left ventricle of the heart as well as improved heart contractility when compared with the control group. This research is particularly significant because the participants in this study were coronary artery disease patients going through rehabilitation, yet they were able to safely improve their health and performance using a HIIT walking protocol (Slordahl et al., 2004).

NEGATIVE RECOVERY

Negative recovery, in a work-to-recovery ratio, refers to a recovery time that is either the same as or slightly less than the amount of time you perform the high-intensity microburst interval. In later chapters, we detail each HIIT protocol to clearly explain the work-to-recovery ratio. To clarify negative recovery here, let's use the example of Tabata. In Tabata training, the ratio is 2:1, meaning that you perform 20 seconds of super-high-intensity movement and then recover for 10 seconds. In the HIIT format known as hard, harder, hardest, a 2:1 ratio consists of 40 seconds of a hard interval followed by 20 seconds of recovery. This is followed by a harder interval (a 30-second work interval with 15 seconds of recovery), and the last, or the hardest, is 20 seconds of the highest intensity followed by 10 seconds of active or passive recovery.

The distinguishing feature of HIIT is this systematic application of the work and recovery bouts, or negative recovery. With negative recovery, oxygen debt (the acute response to physiological overload including breathlessness and fatigue) and ultimately excess postexercise oxygen consumption (EPOC—the long-term response to physiological overload, or the calories that are burned after exercise) follow.

Keep in mind that the first number in the ratio refers to the working phase and the second to the recovery phase. Because the second number is less than the first, the recovery is negative. This is important because without negative recovery, oxygen debt, which is the tired, breathless fatigue you experience when you work really hard during exercise, is difficult to attain.

PHYSIOLOGY OF HIIT

As mentioned, cardiorespiratory adaptations that occur with HIIT protocols are similar, if not superior, to those seen with continuous aerobic activity. But it is important to understand that HIIT protocols are naturally anaerobic; that is, they focus mainly on the fast-twitch muscle fibers (type II) with respect to power development and energy production in the muscles.

Compared to anaerobic metabolism, aerobic metabolism is used primarily during endurance exercise and can continue for longer periods of time by using slow-twitch muscle fibers (type I), aerobic glycolysis, and fatty acid oxidation for energy production. Type I muscles are recruited for lower-intensity, longer-duration activities such as walking, swimming, and cycling and, for some, jogging. During aerobic activity, the body's metabolic needs are met by aerobic metabolism, which uses oxygen to convert nutrients (carbohydrate, fat, and protein) to ATP (adenosine triphosphate) or energy in slow-twitch fibers.

The aerobic system is a bit slower than the anaerobic system because it relies on circulation to transport oxygen to working muscles before creating ATP. When the exercise intensity is aerobic, it is below the lactate threshold or the level at which lactate accumulation does not overwhelm the body's ability to remove it, also referred to as OBLA, or the onset of blood lactate accumulation, and you are able to speak during exercise. However, the further away you get from aerobic activity and the closer you get to anaerobic activity, the closer you get to the lactate threshold, at which point speaking is much more difficult. For example, if you were walking your dog at a comfortable pace, you would be in an aerobic state: contented, but your heart rate is elevated. You may break a sweat, and your body is definitely warmer than it would be at rest. However, if that dog's leash broke and you suddenly found yourself chasing the dog for 10 city blocks, your body would need to make fuel to meet this suddenly much greater energy need. It would do so through the anaerobic energy process. This process is very efficient at creating energy for your muscles at this level of performance, but it also releases chemical by-products that are limiting factors when it comes to exercise performance. When the chemicals (lactate and lactic acid) enter the bloodstream, they change the pH balance of the blood, slow down aerobic enzyme production, and make you feel really tired. This breakpoint where the blood lactate levels rise sharply signifies a significant shift from aerobic to anaerobic energy production. Once the body is unable to clear the lactate, it feels very uncomfortable, and the muscles and lungs may experience burning sensations that make breathing at a controlled rate and continuing exercise more difficult.

ATP is the immediate source of energy for anaerobic muscle contractions, and the necessary anaerobic metabolic processes are produced primarily in the fast-twitch muscle fibers (type II). Although fast-twitch muscle fiber contains only enough ATP to power a few contractions, its ATP pool is continuously replenished by sources of high-energy phosphates to keep this anaerobic supply pool replenished.

During anaerobic activities, the energy is produced in the fast-twitch fibers via the ATP-CP energy pathway (adenosine triphosphate–creatine phosphate), sometimes just called the phosphate system. The pool of creatine phosphate is about 10 times larger than that of ATP, so it serves as a reservoir of ATP, supplying about 10 seconds of energy for short bursts of powerful movements. Unlike the aerobic pathway, this energy pathway doesn't require any oxygen to create ATP. Fast-twitch muscle fibers (type II) are characterized as having a low oxidative capacity and are recruited for rapid, powerful movements such as suddenly standing from a seated position to high-intensity activities such as jumping, throwing, and sprinting. Most of the HIIT exercises we perform recruit fast-twitch fibers and therefore rely on the use and development of the ATP-CP and anaerobic glycolysis energy systems explained here.

The phosphate system first uses all of the ATP stored in the muscles (about 2 to 3 seconds of energy) before moving to creatine phosphate (CP) to resynthesize ATP until that runs out in another 6 to 8 seconds. After all of the available ATP and CP are used up, the body moves on to another anaerobic energy system called glycolysis to continue to create ATP to fuel exercise. Anaerobic glycolysis provides energy via the partial breakdown of glucose, so ATP is created exclusively from carbohydrate; lactic acid is the resulting by-product but it doesn't stop there. Once sufficient oxygen is available, lactic acid is then shuttled into the liver where it is reconverted into glucose through a process called gluconeogenesis. These systems produce enough energy for short, high-intensity bursts of activity lasting no more than a few minutes before OBLA buildup reaches a critical threshold, a physiological marker that occurs when lactate accumulates in greater quantities than can be cleared by the body.

Lactate, a chemical derivative of lactic acid, is formed when sugar is broken down for energy without the presence of oxygen. Sometimes the terms *lactic acid* and *lactate* are used interchangeably, but there is a difference. Lactic acid, which releases a hydrogen ion and binds with a positively charged sodium or potassium ion, forms a salt known as lactate. Lactate production is part of the way the muscles make fuel to work, but the production of lactic acid is a limiting factor in energy production. Burning sensations in the muscles and lungs as well as fatigue make it difficult to move and breathe when blood lactate levels reach critical levels. When the body is nearing the lactate threshold, blood buffers work hard to decrease the lactic acid buildup (called acidosis), but the blood cannot be cleared of the lactate quickly enough. To help clear the lactate, the respiration rate (the rate at which air is pulled into and out of the lungs) increases. As the intensity persists, the body continues to become overwhelmed, experiences blood and muscle acidosis, and then eventually fails because lactic acid reaches a threshold at which it can no longer be absorbed. This is referred to as the lactate threshold.

This technical discussion of the physiology may not seem important to understand because the programs outlined in this book are anaerobic. But since the workouts are 30 to 45 minutes, and up to 60 minutes long, you will also achieve an overall aerobic, cardio training effect that will boost your metabolism and offer you many aerobic health and fitness benefits, too. Table 1.1 summarizes the contributions of energy sources and the approximate duration of those contributions in support of the body's energy systems.

Amplified Aerobic Performance With HIIT

If the preceding information about the research demonstrating the many benefits of anaerobic exercise isn't enough to convince you of the benefits of HIIT, there is

Table 1.1   Anaerobic Energy Availability

Energy system	Duration of contribution
ATP-CP	3-10 seconds
Glucose	60-90 seconds

more. Studies have also discovered an increased mitochondrial density as a result of HIIT, which is considered a major benefit. During aerobic exercise, mitochondria use oxygen to manufacture ATP in a process called cellular respiration, through the breakdown of carbohydrate and fat. In the not-so-distant past, exercise scientists believed that the increase in mitochondrial density (the number of mitochondria in each muscle cell) could occur only with aerobic exercise. However, this is not the case. An increase in the size and number of mitochondria, considered the energy factory of cells, is an expected outcome of HIIT (Giballa, 2009). An increase in mitochondrial oxidative enzymes leads to more effective carbohydrate and fat breakdown for fuel, so an increase in mitochondrial density has a significant impact on energy use, particularly fat use, during exercise. As mitochondria density increases, more energy is made available to working muscles, producing greater force for an extended period of time. For example, because an athlete would be able to run at a higher intensity for longer, more mitochondria equals greater levels of sustained intensity for extended periods of performance.

In the past, it was thought that aerobic activity was the more reliable method for using fat as an energy source. But research conducted in 2008 by Perry and his colleagues revealed that fat burning was significantly higher after 6 weeks of HIIT. This has an important implication for women trying to control their weight through slow, steady-state aerobic activity like walking or running. Unfortunately, the law of diminishing returns implies that the more you apply an exercise stimulus at the same intensity and for the same duration, the more you must continue to do that and more to get the same or similar training result. This is because the body adapts and adjusts to a certain stimulus (intensity) applied consistently over a period of time. The body tries hard to conserve rather than burn extra calories. For example, if I run 3 miles (4.8 km) a day 3 times a week, I may notice weight loss and changes in my ability to sustain that level of intensity for a while, but over time, my body will become accustomed to that stimulus, burn fewer calories, and eventually stop changing. As a result, to challenge my body and achieve the changes I want (lose additional weight), I would have to increase either the duration or the intensity of the run. Shorter, faster runs would improve my performance and burn more calories because of the increased energy cost and overload to the body. Also, the decreased impact forces as a result of less road time would possibly decrease the risk of exercise-related overuse injury and burnout because workouts are shorter.

Shorter Training Times With HIIT

Unlike aerobic exercise, HIIT workouts are performed just below or right at the lactate threshold. The HIIT programs in this book are interval-based training protocols that consist of less than 20 minutes of training time (actually performing the HIIT exercises) in which you use the major muscles of the body in compound movements. You can probably guess that performing such movements is taxing and fatiguing and will result in becoming breathless rather quickly. It is not a surprise that long-duration activities at this level are neither possible nor desired. One of the biggest appeals of HIIT protocols is that the exercise sessions are short, but the results are powerful because the caloric expenditure is greater postexercise. In the 2011 study, researchers discovered that one 6-minute HIIT workout (1-minute warm-up and 4 minutes of HIIT followed by a 1-minute cool-down) burned about 50 calories. However, the subjects' metabolism remained elevated postexercise, and they burned approximately an additional 250 calories in the 24-hour period following. This total of 300 calories burned postexercise is comparable to what people typically burn during 30 minutes of continuous steady-state aerobic exercise (Mylrea, 2011).

EPOC and Oxygen Debt

Reaching the lactate threshold requires short-duration, powerful movements yielding large amounts of reserved energy. The lactate threshold is a physiological marker representing the attainment of oxygen debt acutely and EPOC chronically, two terms to identify the effectiveness of the HIIT exercises presented throughout this book.

Those in the exercise physiology and scientific communities use the term *oxygen debt* in different ways. Regardless of this confusion, it's important to use the terms *oxygen debt* and *EPOC* in our programming because they play an important role in defining perceived exertion and determining the lactate threshold during the HIIT workouts. Let's examine the origins of the concepts of oxygen debt and EPOC and learn the role they play in the HIIT workouts presented here.

After high-intensity exercise or heavy resistance training, the body continues to require and use oxygen at an elevated rate—more so than before the exercise session began. This sustained energy requirement is known as postexercise oxygen consumption, or EPOC. In the early exercise science community, EPOC was referred to as oxygen debt. Researchers A.V. Hill and H. Lupton in 1922 coined this term in reference to a postexercise state and defined it as "the amount of extra oxygen required by muscle tissue to oxidize lactic acid and replenish depleted ATP and Cp (phosphocreatine) following vigorous exercise" (Hill and Lupton, 1923). This definition has actually morphed into EPOC, which describes several events that happen as the body attempts to restore itself to a state of homeostasis, or a postexercise time-out following vigorous exercise sessions. Think of oxygen debt in terms of borrowing money: eventually, you have to pay it back.

During EPOC, the body works hard to restore itself to its preexercise status, or homeostasis, by consuming oxygen at an elevated rate. Homeostasis is an internal state of physiological balance. The disruption of the normal state of the body at rest translates to increased energy usage, or in other words, increased caloric expenditure postexercise.

Because the body continues to expend energy after exercise, EPOC plays a big role in weight management. Research suggests that HIIT has a more pronounced effect on EPOC, or the ability to continue to burn calories postexercise, than aerobic exercise has (Haltom, et al., 1999). One study measured the effects of EPOC on females using heavy resistance during weight training. The researchers concluded that, indeed, a relationship exists between an elevated metabolic rate postexercise and resistance training in the female body. Furthermore, as the weightlifting intensity increased, so did the duration of the EPOC (Osterberg & Melby, 2000).

Postexercise, the body endures much in an effort to return to resting levels. One important activity is cooling the body. HIIT requires much additional energy to return the body to a preexercise core temperature by moving water and waste products to the skin for evaporation and cooling. Another important physiological activity following a HIIT workout is replenishment of the anaerobic energy stores for the phosphagen and glycolyic systems. The body also continues to expend energy to reoxygenate the blood and return circulating epinephrine, norepinephrine, and other hormones back to preexercise resting levels. Energy is also expended to bring the body back to preexercise ventilatory (breathing) and heart rate levels.

In summary, the duration of EPOC is greatest immediately postexercise and declines over a few hours. Some research suggests that EPOC occurs anywhere from 3 to 16 hours postexercise. In one study specifically designed to test for EPOC 16 hours postexercise, participants were found to have elevated and measureable EPOC 38 hours postexercise (Schuenke et al., 2002). It's important to note that the stronger the exercise stimulus is, the longer EPOC effects tend to linger.

For the purpose of this book, we use the term *oxygen debt* to refer to the acute response to high-intensity exercise. For example, when performing the exercises, you will be cued to measure your perceived intensity. Using the rating of perceived exertion scale known as RPE, on a scale of 1 to 10 (1 being rest and 10 being complete exhaustion), our goal is to reach the anaerobic threshold, with a rating that falls between 9 and 10. This is known as oxygen debt and is used as an acute measure or gauge of the immediate response to the exercise stimulus. Achieving EPOC long term is the reason we are attempting to achieve oxygen debt acutely.

What is more remarkable than an exercise protocol in which the time spent training is at least two-thirds less than the time spent in the traditional approach to exercise? That is what HIIT offers and more! The best part of HIIT is that most of the benefits occur during recovery. This translates to working hard, but not as often, and making recovery part of the workout. It may sound too good to be true, but it isn't. The important component to understand is that you need to work really hard when it is required, and allow yourself time to recover when required, so you can reap all the benefits possible without injury or succumbing to overuse or burnout. Although the efforts are high, the benefits are worth it. This book offers the advice you need and the workouts that work to take your fitness to the next level, safely and with maximal effectiveness.

ROLE OF RECOVERY

Exercise by its very design challenges the natural resting state of the body, so recovery is a vital component of the overall fitness program. Adequate postexercise recovery is vital to performance, continued improvement, and a decline in injury risk. This chapter focuses on the scientific principles behind recovery and explains how to apply these principles to determine safe and effective recovery times for your workouts.

Most people who exercise have a strong tendency to focus primarily on the exercise rather than what happens before or after. The reality is that people who exercise spend a much greater proportion of their time in recovery than they do in an actual workout. If the rate of recovery is too short, higher training volumes and intensities are impossible without the detrimental effects of overtraining. In fact, the time we dedicate to appropriate pre- and postexercise recovery may be more important to performance enhancement and injury reduction than the workouts themselves.

High-intensity workouts in particular deliberately damage muscles and other soft tissues, causing short-term destruction in the form of tissue breakdown. Inadequate recovery compromises oxygen and nutrient delivery to working muscles and, coupled with overtraining, decreases the ability to create strength, power, speed, a diminished maximal heart rate, and a lower tolerance to perceived exertion rates. Physiological recovery occurs primarily after exercise and is characterized by the physical efforts of the body's attempt to return to homeostasis. The purpose of a workout is to challenge homeostasis, or the body's normal internal balance. Exercise disrupts homeostasis and, as a result, creates imbalances at the chemical, molecular, and tissue levels. Inflammation is often the result, signaling the immune system to start a process that includes an increase in circulating hormones including adrenaline and cortisol, to minimize the damage and speed up repair. Swelling and muscle soreness complete the response. If a workout is too long or strenuous for the current skill and ability of the exerciser, and recovery is either too short or not allowed, injury and burnout can quickly result.

BENEFITS OF RECOVERY

Recovery is essential to achieving higher training volumes and increases the ability to work at greater intensities without the detrimental effects of overtraining. Recovery normalizes physiological functions (e.g., returning blood pressure to preexercise levels returns the body to resting respiration), stabilizes the cardiac cycle, and returns the heart rate to resting levels. Recovery also restores the cellular environment to a preexercise resting state and is also critical in the reinstatement of energy, including blood glucose and muscle glycogen, two readily available energy sources vital to exercise. Recovery can also trigger an adaptive response. As fitness increases, new blood vessels and muscle fibers grow and flourish and eventually connect to form new neuromuscular pathways. An adapted metabolic response allows higher levels of training, permitting the body to react positively. As long as the overload is progressive, the body can get used to its new need to respond constructively to the increased stressors.

As stated, recovery from training may be even more important that the workout itself, because the repair and rebuilding of damaged muscle tissues and the replacement of needed chemicals can only occur during recovery. Proper recovery minimizes the by-products of the physical stress of workouts. The capacity to recover determines the ability to perform the next workout. It is also provides the emotional and mental renewal necessary to avoid exercise boredom, fatigue, and burnout.

TYPES OF RECOVERY

Optimal recovery is required for each energy system to function at maximal levels. As we learned in chapter 1, adenosine triphosphate (ATP) provides the immediate source of energy for skeletal muscle contraction, but it is limited by the intensity and duration of the exercise. Given that ATP is essential for repeated muscle contraction no matter which energy system is being taxed, you might assume that large stores of ATP are constantly available, but this is not the case.

Energy pathways differ considerably in the maximal available amount of ATP based on the duration for which they can be sustained. When performing anaerobic, powerful movements such as those required in the HIIT workouts in this book, fatigue sets in quickly. During training that requires either of the anaerobic pathways to generate ATP, time and intensity are limiting factors in energy production. Because these high-intensity exercises are frequently repeated over multiple bouts, recovery both in-workout and postworkout is critical.

Let's examine recovery guidelines, keeping in mind that the ratio of recovery time to exercise time is energy system dependent—that is, the type and intensity of exercise dictates the timing and type of recovery the body needs. Recovery is in the form of acute recovery (between training bouts), chronic recovery (between workouts that occur in the same week), and long-term recovery within the training cycle (between training periods). Table 2.1 summarizes the types of recovery.

In-Workout Recovery

For HIIT protocols, the acute phase of recovery is called the in-workout recovery or active recovery. This recovery keeps the body moving and warm, circulates and disseminates accumulated exercise-induced waste products, and gives you a chance to catch your breath and prepare mentally for the next exercise bout. For example, in a Tabata sequence, you might work for 20 seconds and then recover and prepare for the next exercise bout (the next 20-second sequence) during a 10-second in-workout recovery period. Active recovery is really important because it helps to clear blood lactate levels and acidosis between the all-out efforts. This occurs as a result of the deep inhalations and exhalations and slight movements of the body. The muscles act as pumps to clear waste products and bring oxygen and nutrients back to the working muscles. This 10-second period also assists in lowering the heart rate, but it keeps the heart pumping to avoid blood pooling in the lower extremities and maintains the heart rate above minimum and below maximum in preparation for the next 20-second work bout.

Table 2.1 Types of Recovery

Type	Description	Example
In-workout or acute active recovery	Recovery that occurs between training bouts within one workout, or the in-workout recovery phase	20 seconds of exercise followed by 10 seconds of recovery
Chronic recovery—active or passive	Recovery that occurs between workouts during a training week. Active recovery may include a low- to moderate-intensity exercise session between HIIT workouts. Passive recovery may involve manual techniques such as using a foam roller or performing a low-intensity workout.	A HIIT workout requires active recovery for a minimum of 24 hours before the next HIIT workout within a training week. A 20- to 45-minute treadmill walk on an RPE (rating of perceived exertion) scale of 4 to 6 may suffice for active recovery. Using a foam roller for specific muscle work is considered passive recovery.
Long-term recovery	Recovery that occurs within a training phase and may involve a linear or a nonlinear periodization cycle	A planned extended recovery phase between training cycles to allow for recovery from a particular training program or protocol over a period of several weeks or months

In HIIT protocols, the recovery phase of the training ratio is typically negative, which means that the work bout is longer than the recovery bout. For example, in a Tabata protocol, the training ratio is 2:1, meaning that the work phase of the interval is twice as long as the recovery (e.g., a work bout of 20 seconds and a recovery of 10 seconds). The expectation is that the exercise will tax the body's anaerobic energy resources, challenging the Type II muscle fibers (fast-twitch), resulting in oxygen debt and eventually excess postexercise oxygen consumption (EPOC). Becoming breathless is an important part of HIIT because it is the physiological marker that the exercise is a high-intensity stimulus and the body is in oxygen debt.

However, HIIT protocols do not always have to be accompanied by negative recovery bouts. In fact, some HIIT methods use positive recovery, such as for people who may not be able to perform workouts that use negative recovery. A great feature of HIIT is that the ratios can be flipped to meet individual needs. The important point is that whatever ratio is used, consistency is important. For example, if you are using a 1:2 ratio, be sure to stick to it. So if the work bout is 15 seconds, the recovery bout should be 30 seconds. Keeping the ratio consistent throughout a given workout will bring about the physiological effect of breathlessness, and eventually EPOC, a physiological process in which the body continues to expend energy as it repairs itself.

The HIIT workouts in this book typically use the following training ratios, but you can flip them to meet your own needs:

- *1:1 ratio of work to recovery*—30 seconds of work followed by 30 seconds of rest

- *2:1 ratio of work to recovery*—30 seconds of work followed by 15 seconds of rest

- *3:1 ratio of work to recovery*—30 seconds of work followed by 10 seconds of rest

The amount of recovery you need is based on your personal fitness goals, abilities, and needs, which are determined using the guidelines in this book and your own experimentation. Also keep in mind that your ratios may change based on your recovery, the intensity of the exercise, where you are in your periodization cycle, and your ability to perform.

Chronic Recovery

Chronic recovery refers to the time the body takes to recover from a HIIT workout. Think of it as the time between workouts from day to day within a particular week. Additionally, there are two types of chronic recovery—active and passive.

Active Recovery

Active recovery may take the form of a low- to moderate-intensity workout between HIIT sessions. Because HIIT workouts are extremely intense, participating in an active recovery workout the day after a challenging HIIT workout (consecutive HIIT workouts are not recommended) can enable you to continue with intense training without compromising your body through unmanageable overloads, overtraining, or an increased potential for injury. The type and intensity of active recovery depends on you, but guidelines such as the following can help.

Allow Adequate Time Between Workouts

Allow at least 24 hours between HIIT workouts; they are not designed to be performed on consecutive days. For example, if you perform a HIIT workout on Monday, perform the next one on Wednesday or Thursday to allow for adequate recovery.

Don't Neglect Recovery Between Workouts

Recovery workouts do not overload the anaerobic energy systems the way HIIT workouts do; instead, they speed up recovery and repair damaged tissues to create

SIGNS OF OVERTRAINING

Especially when using plyometric (jumping or explosive) exercises in the performance of HIIT workouts, it is always advisable to be aware of signs of overtraining. Overtraining is a condition marked by a failure to adequately recover between workouts, working out too aggressively, performing too many training sessions per week, or not following recommended training and recovery ratios and guidelines.

Overtraining is very common at the onset of a program and after taking time off from exercise, particularly after an illness or an injury. Training plateaus and drops in performance as well as injury and burnout are obvious signs of overtraining. If one or more of the following signs and symptoms occur, training intensity, frequency, or duration should be decreased until they disappear.

- Extreme muscle soreness and stiffness following a training session
- A gradual increase in muscle soreness from one training session to the next
- An unexpected decrease in body weight
- An inability to complete a reasonable training session
- An increase in resting heart rate
- Insomnia
- Injuries to joint tissues, stress fractures, and pain

faster and more powerful muscular units. Exercising at moderate intensity for less than 75 minutes can reduce overall inflammation, increase positive neurotransmitters (such as serotonin and endorphins), stimulate nerve growth, and improve circulation to working muscles and the brain. For example, if you performed a 30- to 45-minute HIIT workout on Monday, on Tuesday you should participate in an aerobic activity (heart rate range at 5 or 6 on a scale of 1 to 10) such as recumbent cycling, using an elliptical trainer, walking or light jogging on a treadmill or outside, or a Pilates or yoga session that focuses on strength, balance, and flexibility as opposed to high-intensity work. Approaching your workouts over the long term with a sense of balance (high-intensity, high-effort workouts separated by lower-intensity workouts) will offer you the best results without setting you up for overuse injuries, inadequate recovery, and eventually, burnout.

Prepare to Begin and Transition Out

Always warm up and cool down before starting any workout, including active and passive recovery workouts. Think of the stress that is put on your car when you are idling and suddenly speed up to 60 mph (97 km/h) in a matter of seconds. This is similar to what your body experiences when you do not perform an appropriate warm-up prior to exercise. Because the purpose of the warm-up is to prepare the body for the upcoming activities, you should view it as a rehearsal as well as physiological preparation. The exercises and movements you select for your warm-up should be dictated by the activity you will be performing. The warm-up should be sufficient to increase core body temperature, lubricate the joints (e.g., shoulders, knees, hips, spinal column) increase blood flow to the major muscles, and increase perspiration.

The cool-down, or the transition out of exercise, should prepare you to move from exercise to rest with minimal compromise. Have you ever stepped into a shower after a hard workout and find you are still sweating? That is evidence that the transition out of exercise was insufficient to bring the heart rate closer to resting levels, decrease blood flow to working muscles, and put the body on notice that the exercise portion of the day is finished. The transition time out of exercise is also a great time to take advantage of warm muscles by performing static, or held, stretches. Because the muscles are warm and pliable, they are more likely to respond to held stretches. You should also take that time to bring your body back to a resting state. Guidelines for a warm-up and cool-down are provided in table 2.2.

Get Enough Sleep

Sleep is the ultimate recovery tool. Proper amounts of sleep allow the body to recover and repair between workouts. Research suggests that 7 to 9 hours of sleep per night is critical for hormonal balance and physical repair. Sleep enhances the muscle-building effect of exercise by increasing protein synthesis, and it helps the nervous system return to a resting state. Sleep boosts immune function, which helps with the recovery of muscle tissue and metabolic balance.

Table 2.2   Warm-Up and Cool-Down Guidelines

	30-minute workout	45-minute workout	60-minute workout
Warm-up	3-5 minutes	5-7 minutes	5-10 minutes
Cool-down	3-5 minutes	5 minutes	5-7 minutes

Passive Recovery

Passive recovery can be thought of in two ways: (1) recovery that occurs immediately following an anaerobic workout or (2) longer-term passive activities that take place between high-intensity exercises sessions. In the first instance, passive recovery occurs immediately following a HIIT interval to replenish ATP-CP stores and remove the waste products that accumulate as a result of high-intensity efforts. Recovery and replenishment of these energy systems is important because they play an integral role in energy production in the next high-intensity interval. Passive recovery may involve lying or sitting down directly after the exercise bout. The disadvantage of passive recovery immediately following an exercise bout is that waste products such as lactic acid and other chemical products are slower to decrease than during active recovery, and blood can pool in the lower body. The advantage is that ATP-CP resynthesis is more rapid; moreover, the longer the recovery time is, the greater the replenishment is. In a Tabata protocol, in-workout recovery time is only 10 seconds long; therefore, it is recommended that you not sit or lie down between HIIT efforts so that you can use the muscles as pumps to avoid blood pooling in your lower extremities. Remaining active also allows for a more rapid removal of accumulated waste products as well as some replenishment of ATP-CP, helps clear waste products, and gets the blood flowing.

A number of techniques can be helpful for passive recovery between workouts to allow the body to return to a resting state. This section discusses in detail the use of a foam roller for passive recovery between HIIT workouts.

The foam roller is an inexpensive piece of exercise equipment. The self-massage technique is also referred to as self-myofascial release, or SMR. The foam roller is used to reach the tissues at the level of the fascia (the encasement of muscles), the tendons, and the ligaments. Rolling can assist in relaxation, releasing muscle knots or adhesions, removing waste products, and generally increasing blood flow and circulation.

Rollers come in a variety of sizes and densities. Thicker, harder rollers feel much more intense than softer, less dense models. Typical rollers are about 3 feet (90 cm) long and 6 inches (15 cm) wide. Some rollers have tread, which can increase the intensity of the experience. Following are general guidelines for performing self-massage with a foam roller:

- Roll about 2 to 3 inches (5 to 8 cm) at a time, avoiding rolling over the joints and bones.
- Roll slowly, maintaining control of the low back and shoulders.
- Be sure to maintain good posture while rolling, engaging the core and stabilizing the spine.
- If a knot or adhesion is felt when rolling, try to release it by holding the body on that point for a few seconds. Mild discomfort should be expected, but not pain. If the knot does not diminish in a few moments, move along and come back to that area another time, maybe on another day.
- If you experience pain, stop rolling. Continuing to roll when pain is present can increase tightness and pain; injury may even result.
- Resting 20 to 30 seconds on painful areas may stimulate relaxation and reduce muscular tension and pain.
- You can roll once or twice daily for as long as you are comfortable.

- Stretch the worked muscles after each rolling session.
- Always drink plenty of water after rolling to assist in flushing out the accumulated waste products and to promote hydration and circulation.

When rolling for self-massage, if you focus primarily on the gluteals, the sides of the thighs or quadriceps, the hip flexors, and the calves, you will get significant relief and will really feel the muscle tightness and tension melt away. Following are instructions for using the roller on a variety of muscles; choose the areas that are best for you.

Piriformis (Deep Gluteal Muscle)

Begin seated on the roller, with one leg bent and your foot on the floor to stabilize the body (see figure *a*). Move a few inches (around 7 cm) back and forth, focusing on the deep muscles of the gluteals and the hips (see figure *b*). Use your hands to help stabilize your upper body.

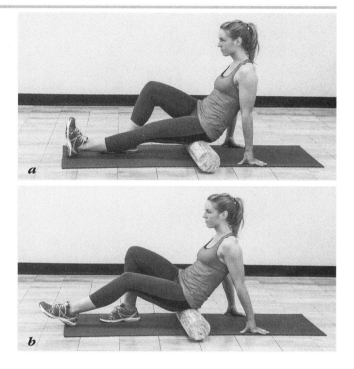

Lateral Hip

Position the upper, lateral hip on the roller. The top leg should be crossed and flexed at the knee, in front of the back leg, which is long and extended (see figure *a*). Roll a few inches (about 7 cm) at a time in a slow, controlled manner, in and around the upper hip and gluteal area (see figure *b*).

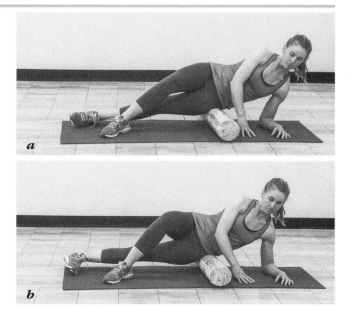

Hip Flexor

Lie facedown on the foam roller with your weight supported with your arms (see figure *a*). Maintain a proper draw-in position while you manipulate the roller over the hip flexor area (see figure *b*). Focus on the muscles that attach your legs to your torso. Do this movement one hip area at a time for best results.

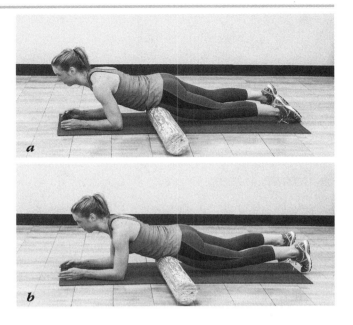

Quadriceps

Position the body facedown with the thighs on the foam roller (see figure *a*). Roll from the pelvic bone to the top of the knee, in sections, to emphasize all the muscle groups of the quads (see figure *b*). You can roll one or both legs at a time.

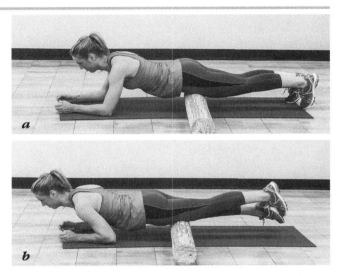

Inner Thigh

Lie facedown with one leg extended wide. Place the foam roller along the inside musculature of the thigh (see figure *a*). Roll in sections over all the areas of the inner-thigh muscle group (see figure *b*).

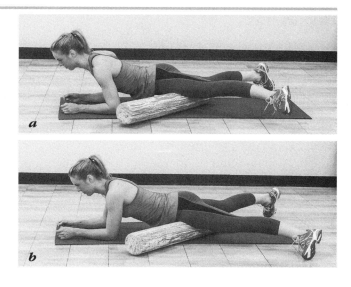

Iliotibial Band (IT Band)

Position yourself on your side lying on the foam roller (see figure *a*). Raise the bottom leg slightly off the floor. Maintain your head in a neutral position with the ears aligned with the shoulders. Roll just below the hip joint and down the side of the thigh to the knee (see figure *b*). You can increase intensity by stacking your legs.

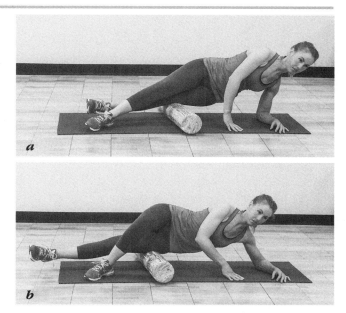

Hamstrings

Sit on the roller with it at the crease between the legs and the gluteals (also called the gluteal fold) (see figure *a*). Begin rolling from the hips down toward the back of the knees, massaging the backs of the legs (see figure *b*). Use your hands and arms to hold your spine upright and to move forward and back. This is a very dense muscular region, so you may need to spend more time here.

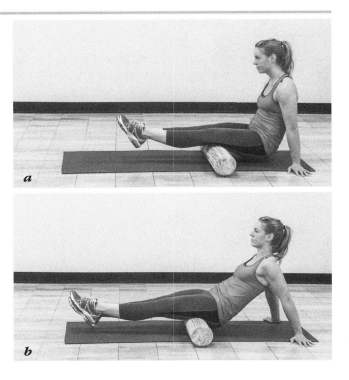

Calves

Prop your body up on your arms, being sure to support yourself while not putting your shoulders into painful positions (see figure *a*). Point and flex your ankle joint as you roll the foam roller up and down the length of the calf (see figure *b*). It is common to get fatigued in the arms, wrists, and shoulders when holding this posture, so take breaks when necessary.

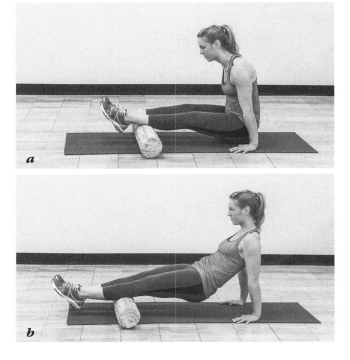

Shins

Stabilize your body on top of the roller (see figure *a*), gently rolling up and down the front of the lower leg and all the way down to the ankle joint (see figure *b*).

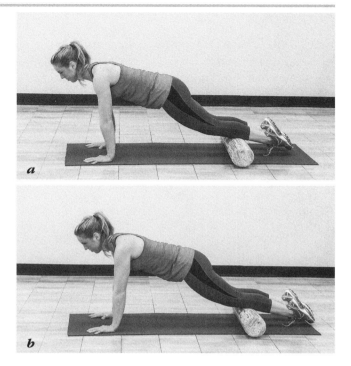

Low Back

Cross your arms and place your hands on opposite shoulders to open the shoulder blades while maintaining an abdominal draw-in position to stabilize the core and spine (engaging the abdominal wall to protect the low back and maintain an upright posture) (see figure *a*). Roll from where your belt crosses your pants down to the lower hip and back (see figure *b*).

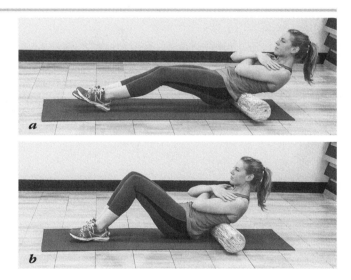

Middle Back

Cross your arms and place your hands on opposite shoulders to open the shoulder blades while maintaining an abdominal draw-in position to stabilize the core and spine, engaging the abdominal wall to protect the low back and maintain an upright posture (see figure *a*). Imagine that you are zipping up a tight pair of pants, but don't hold your breath. Raise your hips until the roller is supporting the middle, upper back (see figure *b*). Be sure to stabilize the head and neck while rolling.

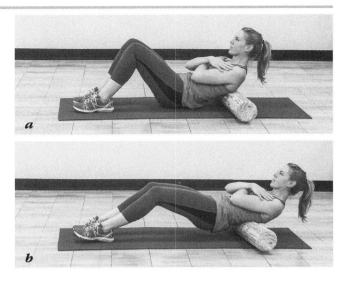

Lats

Position yourself on your side with one arm outstretched and the foam roller alongside the body (see figure *a*). Movement during this rolling sequence is minimal; move the roller along the side of the back, focusing on that area and the lats (see figure *b*).

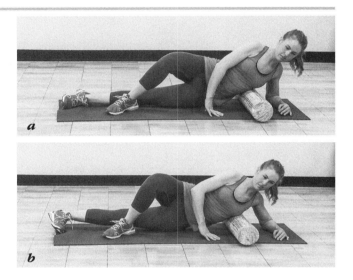

Long-Term Recovery

Your training program should follow a plan and include recovery periods to be well rounded and balanced, decrease your risk of injury and burnout, and help you establish and maintain realistic expectations and goals. Periodization is the systematic approach to planning a fitness training cycle. A periodization cycle is one in which you manipulate intensity and volume to establish a plan that organizes the training into parts or cycles with specific outcome goals. It allows you to plan for increases in intensity and the application of training protocols to achieve specific goals, as well as plan for recovery. Recovery needs to be planned directly into the periodization cycle.

Two types of periodization models can be practical, depending on your goals and your ability to train consistently. Linear periodization is good for exercisers or athletes who have specific goals for their training seasons. For example, a competitive athlete with an in-season, postseason, off-season, and preseason can easily organize training cycles based on the sport. Linear periodization tends to increase in effort and proficiency, followed by a recovery period. A fitness enthusiast using a linear periodization model with a 4-week training cycle may build intensity and volume for 3 weeks and use the fourth week as a recovery week. This pattern can be repeated over several weeks or months, or even up to a year, with tremendous success. Most linear periodization models follow a pattern of decreased training time or repetitions (for strength training) and increased intensity over the course of the training cycle. As an example, table 2.3 shows that during week 1, you perform three 60-minute HIIT workouts with recovery workouts between them. These workouts use a variety of HIIT protocols and degrees of intensity. Week 2 includes two or three 45-minute HIIT workouts that use increased intensity. Week 3 includes two 30-minute HIIT workouts consisting mainly of the highest-intensity HIIT protocols, and week 4 may be dedicated to aerobic recovery workouts only, in preparation for the next 4-week cycle.

A downside to linear periodization is that the highest-intensity training occurs only for a short time during the training cycle. This is probably not an issue for a recreational athlete, but for someone who needs more training volume at the higher intensities and to vary training based on performance goals, linear periodization may be limited. In contrast, nonlinear periodization does not follow a set schedule and does not increase in training volume as the phase continues.

Nonlinear periodization follows a more random pattern and is well suited for exercisers with less ability to plan for exercise and need to exercise around life's uncertainties. Within a given week, you can exercise at higher or lower intensities because the workouts vary from day to day. This could be important because it allows you to work on different skills or at different intensities from workout to workout.

Both linear and nonlinear forms of periodization improve performance, but because everyone responds to recovery differently, you should experiment to discover what works best for you. Table 2.4 provides an example of nonlinear training guidelines over the course of 7 days.

Table 2.3 Linear Periodization Guidelines Over a 4-Week Training Period

Week	Sessions per week	Duration	Difficulty (scale of 1-10)
1	3	60 minutes	7 or 8
2	2 or 3	45 minutes	8 or 9
3	2	30 minutes	9 or 10
4	3-5	45-60 minutes	<7

Table 2.4 Nonlinear Periodization Guidelines Over a 7-Day Training Period

Day	Training focus	Duration
Monday	Maximal power	30 minutes
Tuesday	Upper body and core	45 minutes
Wednesday	Rest	
Thursday	Lower body and core	45 minutes
Friday	Maximal power	30 minutes
Saturday	Core	30 minutes
Sunday	Rest	

Recovery from exercise is essential to performance, but many people still feel guilty about taking a day off from exercise. Rest days are critical to performance from both a physical and psychological point of view. Rest is essential for muscles to repair, rebuild, and strengthen, and the body needs time to return to a state of homeostasis. Building in rest days can help maintain a healthy balance among home, work, and fitness. The next chapters address HIIT protocols, including options you can combine to meet your particular needs and goals.

RECOVERY IS NOT A SUGGESTION

Have you ever experienced an injury as the result of fitness activities, working really hard for extended periods of time, or running long distances day after day without recovery between your runs? If so, you have likely experienced an overuse injury. They are frustrating because they limit your ability to train and interfere with activities of daily living. Overtraining can be very detrimental. Not only can it lead to injury, but it can also result in burnout and have significant long-term negative effects that interfere with a lifestyle of exercise. Fitness and performance enhancement require a complex combination of overload and adequate recovery. Too much overload and too little recovery will likely result in both physical and psychological signs and symptoms of overtraining. Overtraining results from performing exercises that are above and beyond one's tolerance, or beyond the body's ability to recover. Exercising longer and harder without the benefit of recovery will do exactly the opposite of what the training program is designed to do—that is, it will increase the risk and likelihood of injury and decrease performance.

The following signs and symptoms may help you determine whether you are overtraining and not giving yourself enough recovery between workouts:

- Consistent muscle pain and soreness
- Fatigue that doesn't diminish with sleep
- Elevated resting heart rate
- Decline in maximal heart rate
- Insomnia
- Irritability
- Increase in the incidences of illness
- Depression
- Loss of appetite
- Increased incidence of injuries
- Compulsion to exercise
- Loss of enthusiasm for the training or sport
- Drop in performance

You can use your resting heart rate for signs of overtraining. For three consecutive mornings, document your resting heart rate. It should stay relatively consistent from morning to morning. Try to take it at the same time each morning. Any marked increase from the norm may indicate that you aren't fully recovering between workouts. If your resting heart rate begins to rise and you experience other overtraining signs or symptoms, you may be heading into overuse and are likely to experience an injury.

All successful athletes know that rest and recovery between training sessions is critical for optimal, high-level performance. The body strengthens and repairs itself in the time between workouts, and continual training without the benefit of recovery will weaken the strongest athlete. Likewise, fitness enthusiasts need to realize that adequate recovery between workouts is mandatory for reaching their fitness goals without experiencing burnout and increasing their risk of injury. However, many still overtrain, feeling guilty when they take a day off. Rest days are critical to performance. Also, practicing both short- and long-term recovery, as well as planned recovery using periodization, will result in a better balance between lifestyle and fitness goals.

POPULAR HIIT PROTOCOLS

Having examined what HIIT is and how important it is to respect the recovery needs of the body when using HIIT protocols, this chapter explains the differences among HIIT protocols, when to use them, and how to determine which are best to meet your unique needs.

As discussed in chapter 2, recovery is essential to performance over both the short and long haul. Because we differ in fitness levels, goals, and abilities, we need to consider these factors when choosing HIIT protocols in terms of how hard and how long an interval will be, and how much time we will take to recover. The no pain, no gain mentality should not be a factor in work-to-recovery ratio selection. Although it is important to work as hard as you can in any HIIT workout, the ratio needs to match your level of fitness, goals, and abilities. You also need to consider how much recovery to allow, both within and between workouts. Remember that the quality of the movements is more important than the number of repetitions performed; quality should always take priority over quantity.

The following sections examine the popular HIIT protocols. You will learn how to implement these protocols with variety, precision, and appropriate progressions.

TABATA

Although there are several ways to implement HIIT, one of the most popular techniques to date is Tabata training. This 2:1 ratio format, researched in 1996 by Izumi Tabata, consists of 20 seconds of ultra-high-intensity movement followed immediately by 10 seconds of passive recovery. This protocol is performed for 8 rounds, for a total of 4 minutes.

Although this is an amazing training practice with numerous long- and short-term benefits, the average or even above-average exerciser should not be practicing this protocol more than two or three times per week. This protocol is maximal interval training requiring the highest of intensity. Sometimes called a true Tabata, it was designed to be performed on specialized equipment by highly trained, extremely elite athletes. Thus, it should not be used continually over extended periods.

There are ways to take advantage of this 2:1 ratio by using the timing principles of Tabata while avoiding the overuse and overtraining potential of the maximal interval, or true Tabata, experience.

Variations in Tabata timing can be credited to fitness pioneer Mindy Mylrea. Her ideas with respect to the 2:1 Tabata ratio launched a revolution in HIIT training. In Mylrea's formulas, Tabata timing is used, but the intensity of the exercise is increased or decreased based on the movement selection. Exercisers can use Tabata timing ratios without the risk of inappropriate exercise selection or overtraining. The exercise demands are still very high, but because of the exercise selection, the format is very manageable and scalable, even for those at lower fitness levels, at higher risk for injuries, or with other exercise limitations.

Let's examine the different types of Tabata intervals used in this book.

Max Interval

The first Tabata protocol, known as max interval, is most closely aligned with the original 1996 research of Izumi Tabata in that it uses ultra-high-intensity intervals. In a max interval Tabata, a single exercise is performed over eight consecutive rounds using the 2:1 ratio of 20 seconds of work and 10 seconds of rest to absolute failure. This is the most challenging of all the Tabata techniques, because it requires maximal force, power, strength, and speed. Although only one exercise is performed over the course of the 8-round, 4-minute period, the exercise represents the highest, maximal-intensity movement when done with full effort, and it takes the body to the point of performance failure by reaching and crossing the anaerobic threshold quickly. Mylrea has created a checklist that can be very helpful in selecting appropriate exercises for a max interval Tabata. The following sections present guidelines to follow in the selection process.

Use the Entire Body

Because max intervals involve only one exercise, it must address the entire body (i.e., all major muscles). Examples include jump squats, power lunges, and high-knee running in place.

Use Maximal Effort

The exercise in a max interval has to be an immediate hit—that is, it should bring the body to failure quickly. The movement must ramp up in intensity within the first 30 to 90 seconds to allow the body to cross the anaerobic threshold quickly.

Use Simple Movements

Max intervals need to be simple to implement. The exercise's movement sequence needs to be straightforward, because complexity dilutes the intensity by creating confusion. Examples of exercises that are too complex are those that include lead leg changes and those that have intricate movement patterns.

Build Progressions

Max intervals must be scalable. The exercise must have built-in progressions and regressions so that anyone can participate and perform to the best of her ability for the entire 4-minute sequence. For example, a squat could be regressed, or made more accessible, to those with lower levels of fitness by decreasing the range of motion or speed (i.e., creating a built-in off-ramp). Conversely, the same squat can be made more challenging by adding a heel lift or a small or big jump (i.e., offering an on-ramp).

Perform Consistently

Max intervals need to be standardized; the movements must be performed consistently. For example, if the exercise is a squat, with or without a jump, it should have clearly communicated standards to preserve the quality of performance. Standards for the squat might be touching the floor with two fingers each time when lowering down into the squat or reaching the hands straight above the head. These actions must occur with each repetition during each interval.

Mixed Interval

The second training type that follows the 2:1 Tabata timing technique is the mixed interval. A mixed interval offers significant intensity much like a max interval, but somewhat reduced effort during the 4-minute sequence. Mixed intervals offer more variety by combining two or four exercises in the 4-minute Tabata experience. The timing remains the same (2:1 ratio of 20 seconds of work and 10 seconds of rest), but the exercises are organized to vary the training stimulus and can focus on specific body parts. An example of a mixed interval is a combination of jumping jacks and push-ups.

The proper execution of mixed interval sequences is important, because using two or four exercises in the span of 4 minutes with only 10 seconds between them can get confusing. To reduce uncertainty and complexity, which can definitely affect intensity, perform mixed intervals very specifically to avoid misunderstanding and to maintain intensity.

Mixed intervals using jumping jacks and push-ups can be executed using these coaching cues:

Round 1: Jumping Jacks

The performance standard is touching the fingertips in front of the chest each time the feet come together.

Round 2: Jumping Jacks

Be sure the feet come together and the knees track with the second and third toe with each jump in and out. The move can be scaled down by slowing down the jack or stepping out and then in rather than jumping.

Round 3: Push-Ups

Be cautious when moving from an upright position to the floor. The performance standard is to place the right knee on the floor while keeping the arms directly by the sides of the body. Brush the insides of the biceps against the torso with each lowering motion of the push-up.

Round 4: Push-Ups

For this round, place the left knee on the floor for the push-up. Decrease the speed of the movement or the range of motion, or hold the plank at the top of the push-up if the exercise becomes too challenging. However, stopping is not an option.

Round 5: Jumping Jacks

Maintain high intensity even though fatigue is setting in.

Round 6: Jumping Jacks

Maintain the highest effort possible even if fatigue is setting in. Stay consistent with the exercise standards, even if you have to take an off-ramp option (e.g., slowing down) to maintain your intensity.

Round 7: Push-Ups

Make changes to the exercise by modifying the movements to complete each push-up to the best of your ability.

Round 8: Push-Ups

If the intensity becomes too great, take an off-ramp option. For example, put one knee down while performing the down phase of the push-up. Use that same knee (or alternate knees) to help push back up to plank.

As you can see, the moves are ordered consistently to avoid confusion and dilution of the intensity. In this example, rounds 1 and 2 are jumping jacks; rounds 3 and 4 are push-ups; rounds 5 and 6 are jumping jacks again; and rounds 7 and 8 are push-ups again. If performing four exercises, you would simply perform one for round 1, a second for round 2, a third for round 3, and a fourth for round 4, repeating the same sequence for rounds 5 through 8. It is preferable to use two exercises for mixed intervals, because it is easier to remember the exercises. However, sometimes four exercises can add diversity and interest.

Timing Interval

The last Tabata sequence is called a timing interval. This training option is similar to the four-exercise sequence of the mixed interval, but the timing sequence includes four to eight moderately intense exercises as opposed to one, two, or four extremely intense intervals. Timing intervals can offer more options for those with lower fitness levels, those who are just starting out with HIIT formats, or those who are looking for more achievable movements within a Tabata sequence.

The timing technique can also be very useful for a warm-up or cool-down. For example, a warm-up could include four to eight low- to moderate-intensity movements in the Tabata timing ratio of 2:1. The first 20-second round could be a march in place, and the second round could be a side step or a step-touch. The third round could be jumping jacks, and the fourth round might be a squat in place. This sequence could be repeated for rounds 5 through 8, or different exercises could be performed. For the 10 seconds between bouts, easy range-of-motion stretches could assist with the transitions into each new 20-second round. For a cool-down, held static stretches could be performed for rounds 1 through 8 using the 2:1 timing ratio to transition out of the workout. Table 3.1 is a summary of the Tabata methods.

Table 3.1 Tabata Types and Protocols

Tabata interval type	Number of exercises	Protocol
Max interval	1	Eight rounds in the 2:1 ratio of 20 seconds to failure or the highest effort you can make and 10 seconds of passive rest
Mixed interval	2 or 4	Eight rounds in the 2:1 ratio of 20 seconds at a very high-intensity effort and 10 seconds of passive or active rest
Timing interval	4-8	Eight rounds of moderate intensity in the 2:1 ratio of 20 seconds on and 10 seconds of active rest

HARD, HARDER, HARDEST

Another HIIT protocol inspired by Mylrea follows the 2:1 ratio but differs from Tabata in that it progresses in intensity. This training protocol, called hard, harder, hardest, uses one exercise at three intensity, or effort, levels as follows:

- 40 seconds of hard movement, followed by 20 seconds of recovery
- 30 seconds of harder movement, followed by 15 seconds of recovery
- 20 seconds of hardest movement, followed by 10 seconds of recovery
- Repeat

Hard, harder, hardest is very useful in a HIIT workout because it offers significant opportunities for progressions of intensity, with built-in on-ramps to enable you to cross the anaerobic threshold and achieve excess postexercise oxygen consumption (EPOC) by the time you reach the hardest 20-second segment. However, the demands of the movements in the 30- and 40-second rounds are different from those of the 20/10 sequences found in the Tabata formula.

The best exercises to plug into this protocol are those that naturally progress. For example, for the hard segment, simply march in place. Focus on form, arm swing, knee height, foot placement, and core stability. Once the 40 seconds are over, recovery takes place for 20 seconds and can include some easy dynamic stretches in place to prepare for the harder round.

In the harder round, jog in place for 30 seconds. The exercise progresses by just adding intensity through impact and increased speed. The jog in place is harder than simply marching in place, but it offers a built-in on-ramp for intensity. If the jog in place becomes too much, you may return to a march, or try a combination of the two during the 30-second round.

Once the 30-second jogging round is complete, you have 15 seconds to prepare mentally and physically for the hardest round of 20 seconds. This round involves a high-knee jog or run in place. This is the hardest of the three and should involve a full range of motion that takes you over the anaerobic threshold. By the end of this 20-second sequence, you should be breathless. Take 10 seconds to prepare for the next segment of hard, harder, hardest.

THE LITTLE METHOD

In 2009, Jonathan Little and Martin Gibala of McMaster University in Ontario, Canada, created a HIIT protocol now called the Little method. The researchers determined that 60 seconds of high-intensity training (about 95 percent of $\dot{V}O_2max$) should be coupled with 75 seconds of low-intensity training (about 50 percent of $\dot{V}O_2max$) for 12 rounds. This method can be very useful for those who want a HIIT workout but may not want to perform a Tabata workout every time. Additionally, the Little method is easier to progress and regress because you have more time to do so; as such, it is a great option for varying both effort and intensity.

An example of a Little workout is 60 seconds of fast running and 75 seconds of walking for 12 rounds (about 27 minutes). With a warm-up and cool-down of sufficient time, this can be a very time-efficient cardio workout appropriate for people at a variety of fitness levels. Later in this chapter we take a look at MIIT protocols (moderate-intensity interval training); the Little method may be included in this category, depending on the exercises.

FARTLEK TRAINING

Fartlek, Swedish for "speed play," is a fun HIIT option that works well when exercising with a partner or in a group. Fartlek training is also known as discontinuous interval training, because although the recovery is often shorter than the work bout, this is not always the case. Also, the duration of the intervals varies based on a few factors.

Generally, fartlek training is best performed on an indoor or outdoor standard high school track. The easiest method is to have all the participants line up single file. If you have five participants, the first person in line is number 1, followed by number

2, and so on down the line. Participants begin by jogging or walking in a row. At a designated time (e.g., 30 seconds into the walk or jog), the person at the back of the line sprints past the others and is now the front runner. Once she is in place and everyone has established a consistent, rhythmic gait, the person now at the back of the line sprints to the front. This process can go on for a specified distance or time. Because the intervals of sprinting to walking or jogging occur as the line is organized, the new front runner is established, and the person at the back is ready to run, it may not always follow a rigid work ratio, but that is OK. Because the microburst of the sprint to the front of the line is a high-intensity interval, this training modality, although not completely predictable with respect to the ratios, can offer benefits similar to a HIIT session.

MIIT (MODERATE-INTENSITY INTERVAL TRAINING)

With so much emphasis on high-intensity interval training, it is important to understand moderate-intensity interval training and why it continues to play an important role in a well-rounded fitness program. MIIT occurs in mostly the same manner as HIIT, but instead of bouts of super-high-intensity exercise, moderate-intensity intervals are used. For example, on a scale of 1 to 10, a HIIT protocol demands a 9 or a 10 for the hard interval (using the 20/10 format, the 20 seconds would be hard). In the MIIT protocol following the same 20/10 format, the 20 seconds would be a 5 to 7 on a scale of 1 to 10.

MIIT is extremely effective in increasing endurance levels, using fat as an energy source, and taking advantage of the health benefits of exercise without the constant demands of HIIT. MIIT is also great for recovery workouts, which are so important to a well-rounded training program. To avoid overtraining with HIIT, MIIT protocols can be useful in practicing interval training without the overtraining that can accompany HIIT.

HIIT protocols for the purpose of improving fitness and upping the intensity vary greatly. Challenging yourself involves digging a little deeper, pushing yourself a little further than you thought you could go. Simply performing hard workouts can be challenging and difficult, yet they frequently lack planning, progression, and goals based on current skills and abilities. Working hard can set you up to overtrain or become injured, and thus keep you from reaching your fitness goals. HIIT workouts help you to work on the edge without falling off the cliff. They provide results in a safe, creative, responsible way. There is a big difference between working out hard and working out smart. HIIT is called performance-based training for a reason. When training with a performance goal in mind, you do not simply perform difficult tasks mindlessly and without outcome goals. With performance as a goal, fatigue will certainly follow; there's no need to cheapen the experience by just trying to wear yourself down. The methods presented in this book are physically demanding, but always offer on- and off-ramps to ensure movement quality. Standards are designed to assist you in achieving your goals without compromising your health and safety.

INCORPORATING TOOLS AND TOYS

The use of portable fitness equipment in HIIT is a great way to increase the challenge, add variety, and address other elements of fitness such as strength, endurance, and power. Equipment such as medicine balls, stability balls, tubing, suspension trainers, mini-trampolines, gliding disks, kettlebells, and dumbbells can add a dimension to your body-weight workouts. This chapter discusses the safe use and best applications of tools and toys in HIIT workouts.

WHY USE TOOLS AND TOYS?

Often referred to as tools or toys, portable fitness equipment can add much in the way of intensity, variety, stimulus, and focus on specific body parts to HIIT workouts. Although it is imperative that body mechanics, free of any equipment, is the primary focus during any HIIT sequence, equipment can add interest and fun. For example, medicine balls can add a new dimension to building endurance and strength in the upper body. Stability balls can offer a unique experience for the push-up; being off the floor offers a different type of upper-body and core challenge. Tubing can add a fresh aspect to resistance training for a particular body part. All of these tools are relatively lightweight, portable, and easy to use and store, and they can add much in the way of concentration and challenge while training.

If you don't have these tools or toys, you can still perform HIIT workouts by using body-weight exercises; tools are not required. However, they can provide an assortment of options and the variety you may want or need to achieve a specific training goal.

TOOL AND TOY SAFETY

When using equipment during HIIT workouts, safety must be your first priority. How you use the equipment is an important consideration. Tools and toys should facilitate the experience, not take away from it. If they are not making the exercise more effective or adding a unique challenge, they may not be helpful. Because HIIT protocols can be extremely physically demanding with high-impact and lateral and forward movements, equipment that is lying around may become a distraction or a danger. When using portable equipment, make sure to place it out of the way of your moving body to avoid stepping on it or tripping over it.

Following is a list of key points for the safe use of tools and toys:

- Have an understanding of your personal goals, skills, and abilities, including any previous injuries or personal limitations.
- Choose weights or loads that you can control completely at all times.
- Read instructions regarding the proper usage of and weight restrictions for tools and toys such as stability balls and suspension trainers.
- Place all equipment out of the way of moving bodies when not in use.
- To avoid slipping or dropping equipment, wipe down equipment that gets wet from sweat.

TOOL AND TOY OPTIONS

Of the many tools and toys that can be used during HIIT workouts, it's important to figure out which are best for you based on your fitness goals and interests as well as what you have available. The following sections address a variety of toys and tools that can be used during HIIT workouts, including size and weight recommendations and what they are best suited for.

Medicine Balls

Medicine balls are used for upper-body pushing and pulling movements and endurance or strength-based core exercises and rotational movements. They also add load to the lower body during squats or lunges or during throwing. Lightweight medicine balls are optimal; stick with 2-, 4-, 6-, or 8-pound balls (between 1 and 4 kg).

Stability Balls

Stability balls provide support and challenge during upper- and lower-body exercises. They also provide added resistance and stability challenge for core exercises. Burst-resistant balls that are 55 or 65 cm (22 or 26 in.) are recommended.

Resistance Tubing

Resistance tubing provides a multiplanar strength and endurance challenge and can be used for upper- or lower-body exercises. In addition, core stability training almost always plays a role when using the resistance tubing. Using the tubing in a variety of ways can mimic real-life movements, thus adding to the functional aspect of training.

Tubing can be long with handles or in a figure-eight shape. The resistance changes with the length of the tubing as well as the thickness. Color usually indicates the degree of resistance.

Suspension Trainer

A suspension trainer provides a unique way to train the upper body, lower body, and core. Once anchored, the suspension trainer adds cardio, strength, flexibility, and endurance challenges to a HIIT workout. Suspension training takes advantage of gravity and the placement of the body relative to the anchor point. Several brands of suspension trainers are available, but TRX suspension trainers are the most popular and are commonly used for body-weight training. Suspension trainers have a steeper learning curve and require more instruction than the other tools and toys, but they are easily adopted and quickly mastered.

Mini-Trampolines

Personal fitness trampolines, or mini-trampolines are a great option for high-intensity interval training because they take away much of the ground reaction forces during high-impact jumping, but still allow for significant intensity and challenge. Many trampolines on the market can support up to 350 pounds (159 kg) of body weight and come in both spring-loaded and cord-attached models.

Proper technique is important when using trampolines during HIIT workouts to get the proper exercise stimulus to cross over the anaerobic threshold. For example, it is important to learn how to push down, or load down, when using the trampolines as opposed to jumping up.

Gliding Disks

Gliding disks are small plastic or cloth disks that slide across the floor. They can add intensity and challenge to just about any exercise for the upper body, lower body, or core, such as jumping jacks, lunges, and push-ups.

The disks are about the size of a paper plate and slide easily across the floor when pressure is applied appropriately. Towels or paper plates can be substituted for gliding disks. Towels are best to use on wood surfaces; and paper plates, on carpeted surfaces.

Kettlebells

Lightweight kettlebells are an excellent stimulus for building strength, endurance, and power; controlling rotation; and moving through multidimensional planes. Kettlebells are great for increasing grip strength and controlling momentum, which requires significant core commitment and total-body engagement.

Because kettlebells are swung, only one is necessary. The body responds differently to a kettlebell than it does to a dumbbell with respect to controlling the joints and engaging the muscles of the core. Because of the fast-paced environment of HIIT, lightweight kettlebells are strongly recommended: 4, 6, 8, 10, 12, and 15 pounds (between 2 and 6 kg).

Dumbbells

Dumbbells help increase strength, stamina, endurance, definition, and tone in working muscles and can add significant load to exercises within a HIIT routine. Dumbbells are a safe and effective way to incorporate strength training with a cardio workout. Be sure to use weights you can control; 8-, 10-, 12-, 15-, and 20-pound (between 4 and 9 kg) weights are best for this type of training.

Toys, tools, and other portable equipment can be very useful in HIIT workouts because they offer variety and additional challenge. They can also be extremely effective because the dynamic movement patterns can add significantly to the HIIT programming outcomes and overall exercise experience. Tools and toys also allow you to focus on particular body parts for increased endurance, better muscle tone and development, and improved strength while performing HIIT.

The next chapters explore the application of these tools and toys and present exercises that incinerate fat, shape and tone the upper and lower body, improve core strength to improve posture and enhance exercise performance, and strengthen muscles to improve movement and balance.

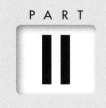

PART

II

HIGH-INTENSITY
INTERVAL EXERCISES

LOWER-BODY EXERCISES

The human body is capable of a variety of movements, but some exercises work best for the HIIT workouts, depending on the type you are performing. Even though only a finite number of movements can be selected for any exercise program, the variations of moves are never-ending. And although tools and toys are available for HIIT exercises, the least expensive and most readily available piece of equipment is your own body. Body-weight exercises are extremely effective and best suited for HIIT protocols. The key is to choose them based on your outcome goals. Also, it is important to understand exactly what the exercise should look like, how it should be performed, and what corrections should be made to create movement patterns that are safe, effective, and progressive.

LOWER-BODY MUSCLES

The lower-body musculature consists of the thighs, also known as the quadriceps, the hamstrings, the gluteals or hips, the adductors or inner thighs, and the calves. The gluteal muscles extend the hips and move the legs back and away from the body. They also work to lift the legs out and to the side of the body, as in side leg lifts. The adductors, or inner thighs, move the legs back in toward the midline of the body. The hamstrings, located on the posterior, or back, of the thighs, flex the knee joints and move the heels up toward the hips. The quadriceps, located on the front, or anterior, thighs, extend the knee joints, straightening and lifting the legs. The calves assist the knees and point the ankle joints downward (plantar flexion) as well as help raise the body up onto the toes. All of these movement patterns are performed in the course of the lower-body exercises you will do as part of your HIIT workouts. See figure 5.1 for an illustration of the lower-body muscles.

Whether using body weight, tools, or toys, and depending on the area of the body you are targeting, some moves are better for your particular skills, ability, and goals than others. An awareness of the muscles that comprise the lower body will help you select the right exercises according to your outcome goals and give you a better understanding of what the muscular focus should be. The following sections present the best lower-body exercises for HIIT programming, discuss the importance of using plyometrics, and describe the foundational movements using body weight.

Strong lower-body muscles are important for everyday, functional activity including walking, running, climbing stairs, and even sitting down and standing back up again. Because the lower body is the base of support for the entire body, including

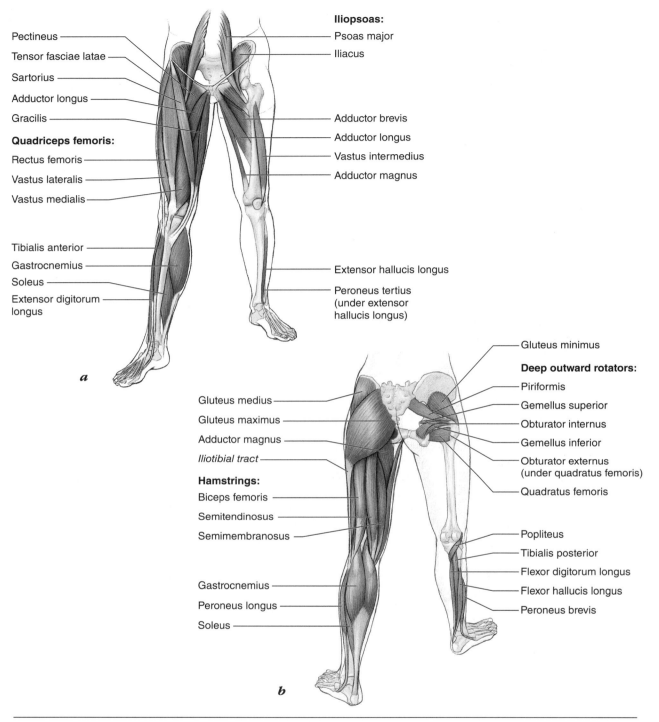

Pectineus

Tensor fasciae latae

Sartorius

Adductor longus

Gracilis

Quadriceps femoris:

Rectus femoris

Vastus lateralis

Vastus medialis

Tibialis anterior

Gastrocnemius

Soleus

Extensor digitorum
longus

Iliopsoas:

Psoas major

Iliacus

Adductor brevis

Adductor longus

Vastus intermedius

Adductor magnus

Extensor hallucis longus

Peroneus tertius
(under extensor
hallucis longus)

a

Gluteus medius

Gluteus maximus

Adductor magnus

Iliotibial tract

Hamstrings:

Biceps femoris

Semitendinosus

Semimembranosus

Gastrocnemius

Peroneus longus

Soleus

Gluteus minimus

Deep outward rotators:

Piriformis

Gemellus superior

Obturator internus

Gemellus inferior

Obturator externus
(under quadratus femoris)

Quadratus femoris

Popliteus

Tibialis posterior

Flexor digitorum longus

Flexor hallucis longus

Peroneus brevis

b

Figure 5.1 The lower-body muscles: *(a)* anterior view and *(b)* posterior view.

the spine, the upper body, and the head, lower-body strength is critical for balance, support, and stability in the rest of the body. Additionally, because the largest muscles are located in the lower body, work in this area burns a substantial number of calories and increases lean mass and metabolic activity. Coordinated and balanced lower-body strength is important to exercise performance and overall health and fitness.

Also, lower-body strength is critical for performing intense physical activity, including jumping, squatting, lunging, running, and hopping, all of which are used in HIIT workouts. Because the muscles of the lower body are the largest in the body, they are critical for creating in-workout oxygen debt.

HIP HINGE

The hips are really essential in power development and low back protection when performing lower-body movements. Using the large muscles of the hips and protecting the back are key when performing any exercise, but particularly lower-body exercises. The hip hinge is the fundamental movement pattern for many of the lower-body exercises presented here. If the hinge is not done correctly, the exercise using the hinge is compromised.

A hip hinge is flexion originating at the hips (where the legs attach to the torso), with extension of the spine, meaning that it is lifted, upright, and elongated. In a correctly executed hip hinge, muscle tension shifts into the posterior core; tension develops in the gluteals, hamstrings, and back; and weight is firmly rooted throughout both feet. A hip hinge is not the same as a squat, rather it is part of the squat motion.

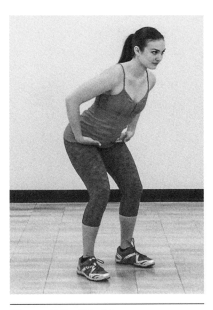

Figure 5.2 Hip hinge.

To perform a hip hinge, stand with feet hip- or shoulder-width apart, toes turned somewhat out. Sit slightly back, and bend first at the hips and then at the knee joints (see figure 5.2). You should have maximal flexion at the hips with minimal flexion at the knees. The knees bend only slightly, while the spine is erect, and the pelvis shifts into an anterior tilt. Lower the hips down and drop the hips and tailbone simultaneously, pushing the butt back. I often use the cue "hand sandwiches" to help people create the proper hip hinge. Place your hands, palms faceup, in the fold between where your legs attach to your body and your lower abdomen. As you hinge, your hands should get stuck in that space. If you are hinging incorrectly, your hands will move easily in and out of that hip fold. If that is the case, you are likely rounding your back as opposed to extending it.

FOUNDATIONAL MOVEMENTS FOR THE LOWER BODY

Foundational movements are standardized body-weight exercises based on the ability to move in specific joint ranges of motion in specific planes of motion. For example, a squat is a foundational movement for the lower body. But a basic squat can look very different based on outcome and training goals. Performing a squat with a kettlebell or gliding disks or simply adding a vertical jump changes the exercise, offering more options for HIIT workouts.

Following are descriptions of foundational lower-body exercises that can be used in HIIT workouts, including how to execute them at the most basic level as well as additional options. Chapter 8 describes many exercise sequence options.

Foundational Movement 1: Squats

To use squats as part of a HIIT program, you need to understand why they are done and how to perform them. Squats are foundational moves because they are part of everyday activities in which body weight is evenly distributed through both feet (e.g., bending down to pick something up off the floor, lowering into a chair or onto a toilet seat). Additionally, because squats require a significant contribution of lower-body muscle and joint action, they can use a lot of energy. Therefore, a variety of squats are presented to help you achieve appropriate overload in your HIIT workouts.

Basic Squat

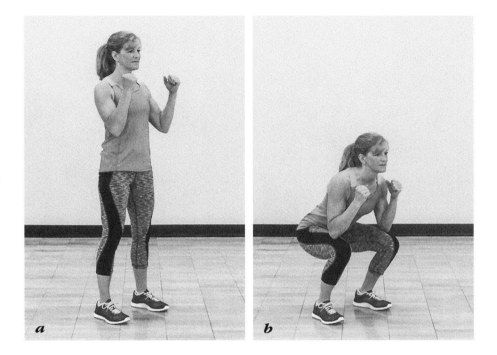

Stand with feet parallel and slightly wider than hip width and toes turned slightly out (see figure *a*). Maintaining an erect spine, lower the tailbone down toward the floor, pressing the hips back and maintaining a neutral neck with the chin parallel to the floor (see figure *b*). The knees may or may not pass the foot, but they should track with the second and third toe of each foot. Flex the knees and lower the body down as low as you can while keeping an erect spine without feeling any pain in any joint, including the knees and hips. The goal is to get the thighs parallel to the floor, while distributing your weight evenly between both feet. You will have a maximal hip hinge here. When you are ready, press through the feet back up to a full upright stance.

Squat to Heel Raise

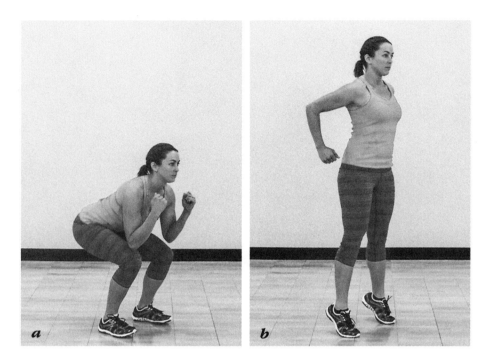

Stand with feet parallel and slightly wider than hip width and toes turned slightly out. Maintaining an erect spine, lower the tailbone down toward the floor, pressing the hips back and maintaining a neutral neck with your chin parallel to the floor (see figure *a*). Rise to an upright stance and continue the movement by rising onto the balls of the feet, lifting the heels off the floor (see figure *b*). Be sure to stay aligned in the foot when lifting the heels and balancing on the balls of the feet; do not drop the heels out or in.

Squat Jump

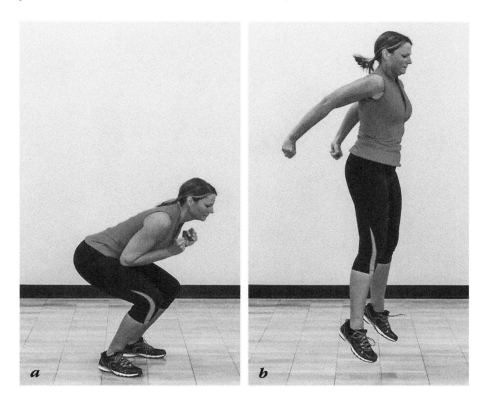

Stand with feet parallel and slightly wider than hip width and toes turned slightly out. Maintaining an erect spine, lower the tailbone down toward the floor, pressing the hips back and maintaining a neutral neck with your chin parallel to the floor (see figure *a*). Rise up to an upright stance, and add a power move by jumping straight up (see figure *b*). Land softly and immediately lower back down into the squat and repeat.

Squat With Elbow Drive

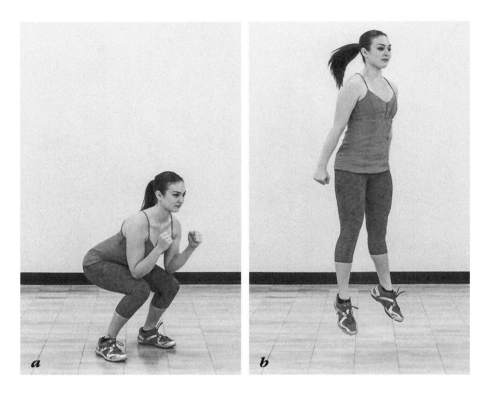

Stand with feet parallel and slightly wider than hip width and toes turned slightly out. Maintaining an erect spine, lower the tailbone down toward the floor, pressing the hips back and maintaining a neutral neck with your chin parallel to the floor (see figure *a*). Rise to an upright stance, and add a power move by jumping straight up and driving the elbows back (see figure *b*). Land softly, immediately lowering back down into the squat and keeping the forearms parallel as you bring the elbows down, touching elbows to the tops of the thighs. Use this elbow-to-thigh movement to standardize the squat and control for quality. Repeat as prescribed.

Offset Stance Squat

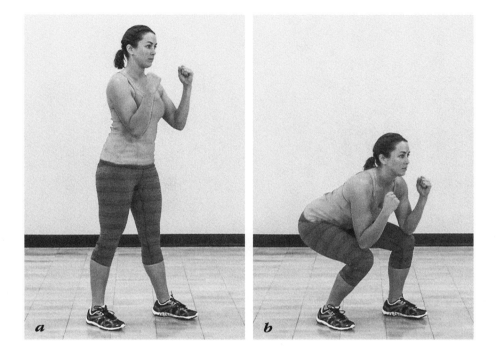

Stand with one foot slightly in front of the other and the feet at least hip-width apart (see figure *a*). Imagine standing on two railroad tracks with your back foot at a slight 45-degree angle and the front foot facing forward. Lower your body into a squat position, keeping the weight evenly distributed between both feet (see figure *b*). Avoid lifting the back foot by keeping your back heel down, loading weight into the entire foot. Intensity can be increased by adding a jump or a heel raise to the squat. Perform as many squats as prescribed, and then switch the lead (front) foot.

▶ Single-Leg Squat

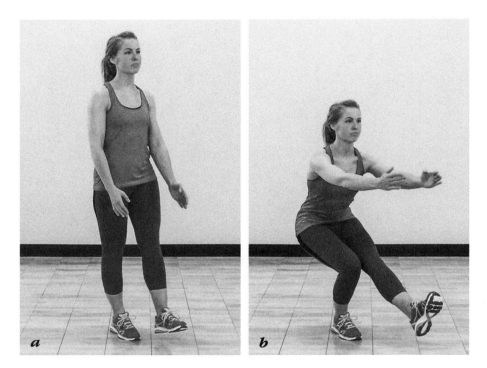

Stand so you are balancing on one leg (see figure *a*). Squat down as far as possible with the other leg extended in front and as high as you can hold it (see figure *b*). Keep your spine as straight and upright as possible. Keep the knee of the supporting leg tracking with the toes of the grounded foot. If you are performing this single-leg squat properly, your extended leg will fall slightly below the flexed knee as you lower into the squat. Rise back to an upright standing position and repeat.

Quarter-Turn Squat

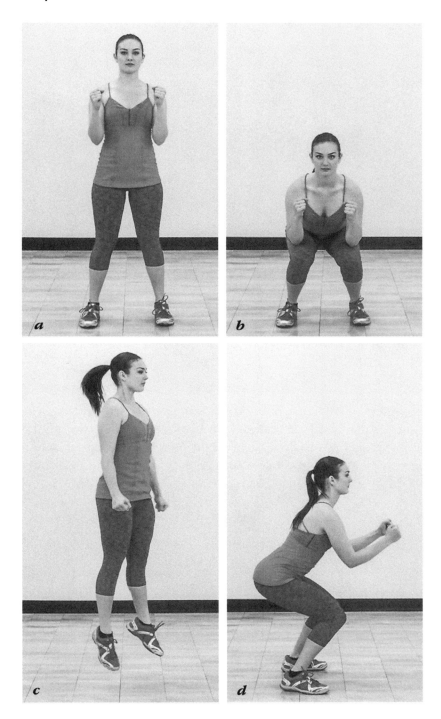

Stand with feet parallel and slightly wider than hip width and toes turned slightly out (see figure *a*). Maintaining an erect spine, lower the tailbone down toward the floor, pressing the hips back and maintaining a neutral neck with your chin parallel to the floor (see figure *b*). Rise back to upright, jump up, and make a quarter turn into a squat (see figure *c* and *d*). Repeat the squat and continue to include the quarter turn with the power jump. If you start to feel dizzy from the turning, just maintain the squat jump or perform the quarter turns by alternating to the right and left.

Side-to-Side Squat

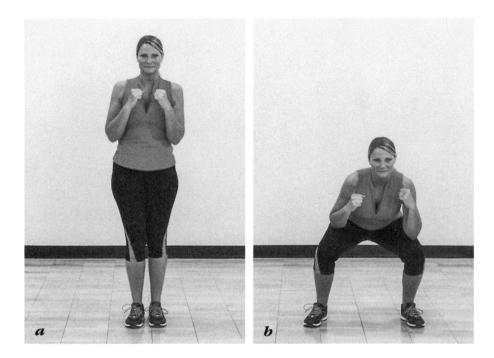

Stand with your feet parallel (see figure *a*) and take a big step out to the side, lowering your body into a squat and flexing both knees (see figure *b*). Lower until your thighs are as close to parallel to the floor as possible. Rise back to upright and simultaneously push off from your foot using your hips and gluteals and return to an upright posture. Repeat by alternating lead legs.

Plié Squat

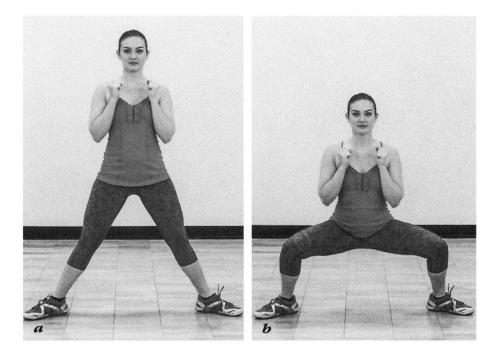

Stand with feet wider than hip width and toes turned out until you can feel the contraction in the gluteal muscles (see figure *a*). Keep the spine very upright as you lower the tailbone vertically toward the floor (see figure *b*). Keep your weight evenly distributed between both feet, and track your knees over the second and third toes of each foot. Return to an upright stance by straightening the legs and repeat.

▶ Plié Squat With Heel Click

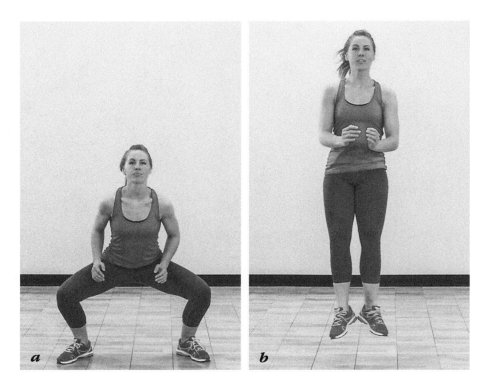

Stand with feet wider than hip width and toes turned out until you can feel the contraction in the gluteal muscles. Keep the spine very upright as you lower the tailbone vertically toward the floor (see figure *a*). Rise to an upright stance, and jump up and off the floor, clicking the heels together in the air (see figure *b*). Land softly with feet hip-width apart, immediately lowering back into the plié squat and repeat.

Squat Jack

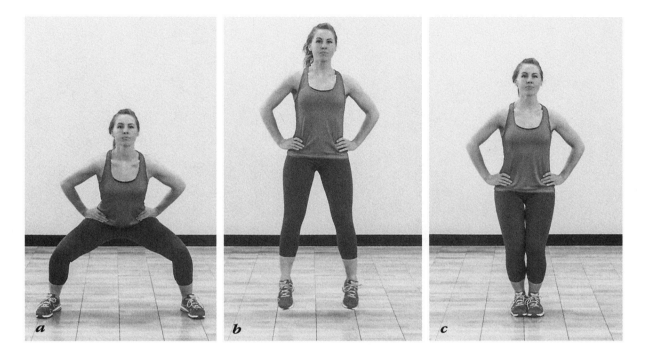

Begin with feet together and then jump out into a wide squat stance as if performing the jump-out phase of a jumping jack but much slower. When you jump out, lower into a squat and hold until you feel stable (see figure *a*). Return to the starting position with a jump into the upright standing posture (see figure *b* and *c*). This exercise may be performed faster or slower based on your goals and ability to stabilize.

▶ Wood Chop Squat

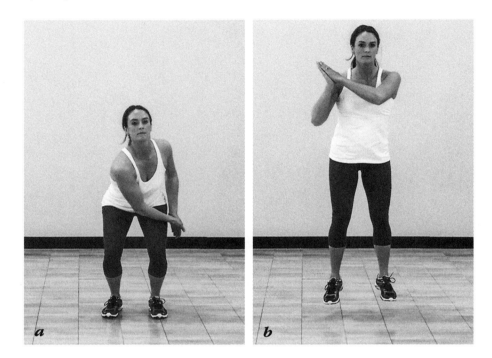

Stand with your feet wider than hip width, and bring your hands together in prayer position up close to and in front of your right shoulder. Lower into a squat position and bring the arms (with hands pressed together in prayer position) down to the outside of the left knee, turning the torso or rotating the spine as little as possible (see figure *a*). Continue to lower and raise the hands from the shoulders down to the knees, adding power to the squat to increase intensity (see figure *b*). Perform as many as prescribed, and then change sides.

Burpee

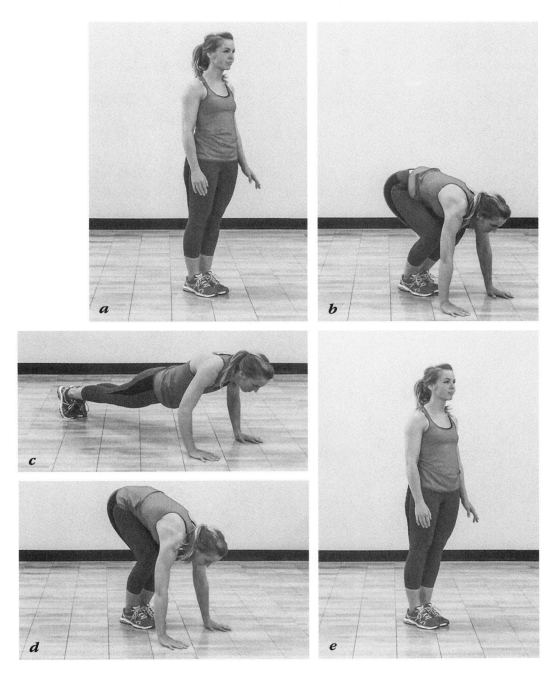

From a standing position with feet hip-width apart or even closer (see figure *a*), lower into a deep squat, bringing the hands to the floor and placing them on either side of the feet (see figure *b*). Keep the feet together and jump back and out to a push-up position, holding the body in a plank (see figure *c*). Then immediately jump the feet back in toward the hands (see figure *d*) and come back upright, returning to a standing position (see figure *e*). Repeat. For more intensity, add a push-up and a vertical jump.

Foundational Movement 2: Lunges

As with squats, everyday life is filled with lunging actions from walking and running to climbing stairs and getting in and out of a car. In each of these activities, your feet are in different lines, at different angles, in a variety of planes of motion, and sometimes at different heights. For this reason, it is important to train the muscles and movements that stabilize the spine and other joints during these motions. Unlike in a squat, in a lunge the body weight is not distributed evenly through both feet. You need to be aware of your weight distribution to ensure proper execution of lunging movements. Lunges also involve several of the major lower-body muscles and occur in a variety of planes of motion. Also, because of the many movements that include lunges, they are performed in a number of ways.

Basic Lunge

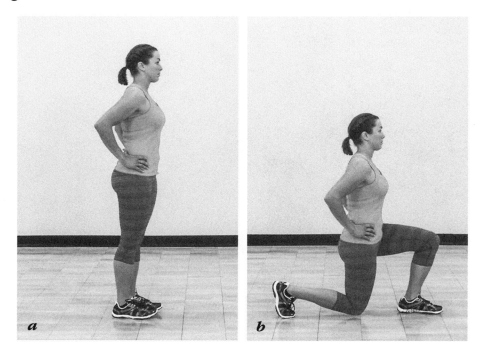

From a standing position (see figure *a*), take a giant step forward, bending at the knee of the front leg and lowering yourself until your front thigh is parallel to the floor (see figure *b*). Your weight will be loaded into the front foot and back forefoot. The back heel will lift off the floor. Your weight should be distributed between the ball of the back foot and the entire front foot. Stay upright through the spine, as if you were balancing a plate on your head. From a side view, your ear, shoulder, hip, knee, and ankle bone should align over the front ankle.

Front to Back Lunge

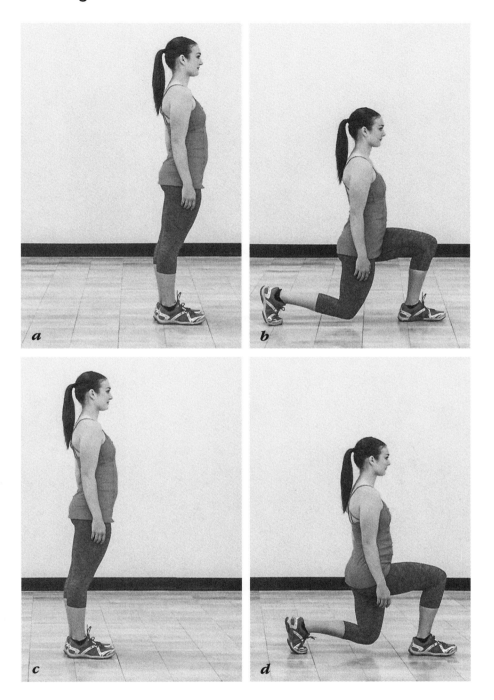

From a standing position (see figure *a*), take a giant step backward with the right leg, lowering your body until the right knee almost touches the floor and the thigh is vertical and under the hip (see figure *b*). Make sure the front knee tracks over the front ankle or foot. Push off the back foot and return to a standing position (see figure *c*). Now, take a giant step forward with the right leg, lowering your body until the left knee almost touches the floor (see figure *d*). Switch legs and repeat.

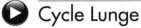 Cycle Lunge

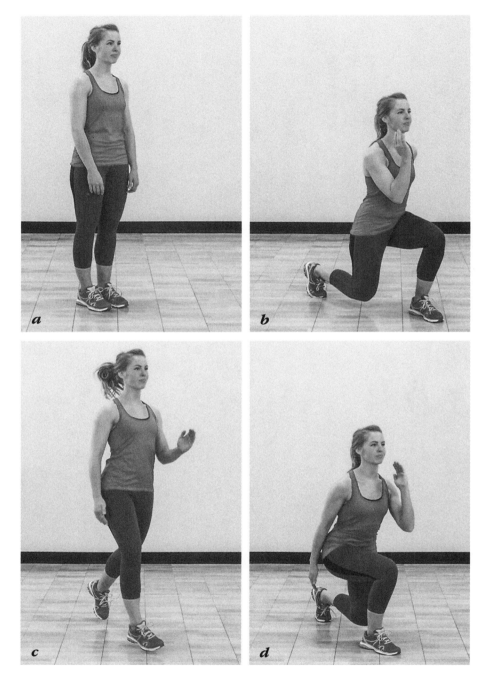

Stand upright (see figure *a*) and take a giant step forward with your left leg, stepping into a front lunge (see figure *b*). Lower into the lunge, and with a big jump up, move vertically and switch the legs in midair (see figure *c*) so that the right leg and foot are in front and the left leg and foot are in back (see figure *d*). Continue this alternating power move focusing on the vertical component. Take as much time as you need to make sure the back knee drops to the floor, directly below the back hip, and the front knee flexes over the front ankle and foot. Continue to alternate as prescribed.

Diagonal Lunge With Floor Touch

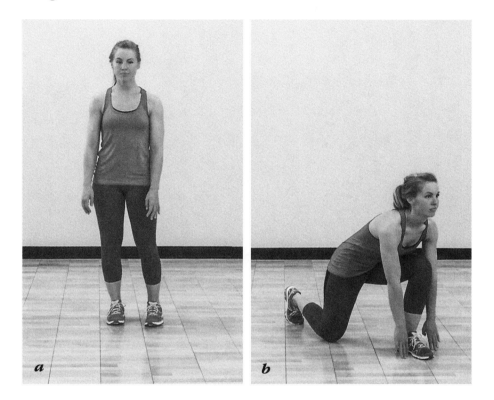

Begin by standing upright (see figure *a*) and step forward into a front lunge and touch the floor directly to the sides of the front foot. Keeping the spine as upright as possible, hinge at the hips as you flex forward (see figure *b*). Step back to an upright stance with feet parallel, and repeat with the other leg.

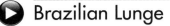

Brazilian Lunge

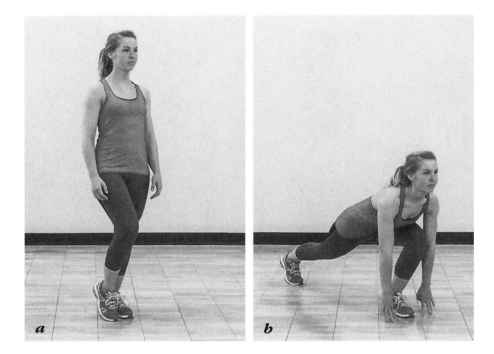

Begin standing upright (see figure *a*) and lower into a runner's lunge by placing the left foot directly under the left, flexed knee and placing both hands lightly on either side of the front foot, with as little weight as possible in the hands and fingertips (see figure *b*). The back leg is extended with the knee straight and the hamstring lifted as high as possible. Use the back foot to step in, placing the feet parallel to each other, and rise to an upright stance. Step back again with the right leg, lowering to the starting position, and repeat. The intensity can be increased by adding a knee lift or a single-leg hop. Repeat on the same lead leg as prescribed, and then switch legs.

Messy Lunge

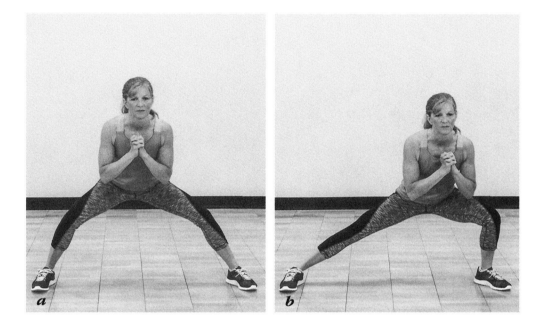

Step with feet wide, toes turned slightly out, and knees tracking over the second and third toes of each foot (see figure *a*). Lower the body and flex the left knee while the right leg stays straight and extended at the knee. Hinge at the hips and maintain an erect spine, keeping the chin parallel with the floor (see figure *b*). Shift your body weight from side to side, minimizing the vertical displacement (i.e., stay low and try not to bob up and down as you slide the body weight from one leg to the next). Alternate the lead from the left to the right. As you move to the side, allow the knee to flex as the opposite leg lengthens, and continue to alternate this movement sequence, keeping the tension in the lower body, legs, and hips.

▶ Single-Leg Balance Lunge

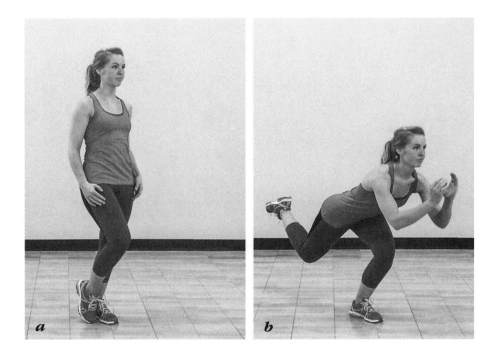

Begin by standing on one foot with the supporting leg straight, flexing the opposite knee so the foot hangs in the air behind the body at knee height (see figure *a*). Lower the body toward the floor, flexing the supporting leg and continuing to balance on the supporting leg (see figure *b*). Attempt to get the back flexed knee as close to the floor as possible. Continue to stabilize and balance; then slowly return to an upright posture. Stay with the same lead leg until it is time to switch legs.

Curtsy Lunge

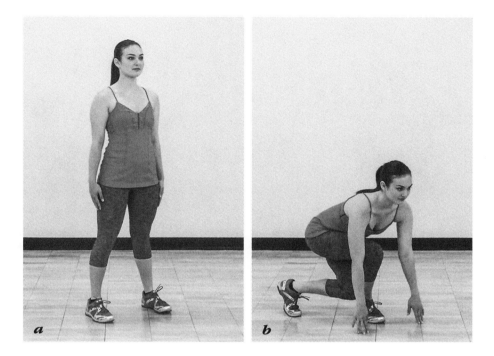

Begin with feet parallel and hip-width apart and toes forward (see figure *a*). Lower onto your right foot, keeping weight in the foot and tension in the muscles of that supporting leg. Use your left leg to step back and to the side, placing the ball of your left foot on the floor slightly behind and to the side of the body. Lower yourself until the front thigh is as close to parallel to the floor as possible, with maximal hinge at the hips and flexion in the knees (see figure *b*). Stabilize the spine by drawing the abdominal wall in and bracing the core; then rise back up to standing, replacing the left foot back to parallel. Repeat on the other leg.

Lateral Lunge With Touch

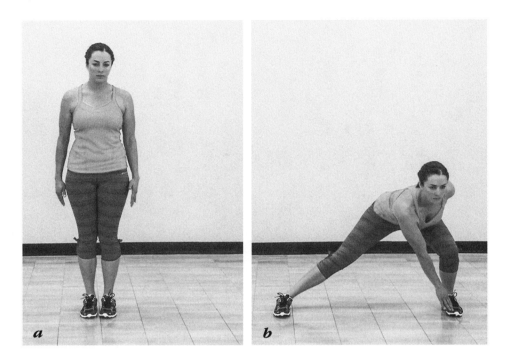

Begin with feet together and a tall, extended spine (see figure *a*). With your left foot, take a large step out to the side, stepping wide and lowering yourself with a maximal hinge in your hips. Flex your left knee, but keep your right leg straight and drive your hips back. Keeping the spine extended, flex the neck (tuck the chin) and focus your eyes on the floor about 2 to 3 feet (60 to 90 cm) in front of you. With your fingertips, touch the left foot (see figure *b*). Return to an upright position by driving through the hip as you push through your foot and leg.

Lateral Lunge With Adduction

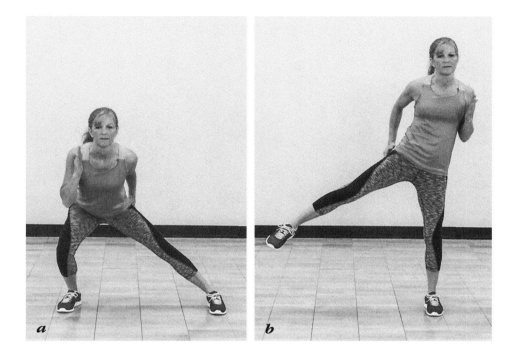

Begin by standing with feet hip-width apart with a tall, extended spine. With your right foot, take a large step out to the side, stepping wide and lowering down toward the floor with a maximal hinge in your hips (see figure *a*). Flexing your right knee and keeping the left leg straight, drive your hips back and keep your spine extended. Tuck your chin and focus on the floor about 2 to 3 feet (60 to 90 cm) in front of you. As you return to an upright posture, drive up with power and lift the right leg straight out to the side (see figure *b*), and then lower it back down, flexing the knee again and loading weight back into the foot and hip.

▶ Front Lunge With Knee Lift

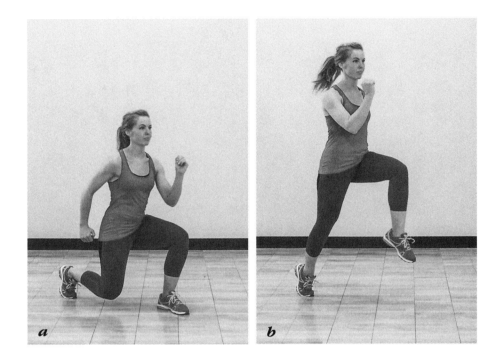

Begin by standing in a wide, split stance; the left foot is in front and the right leg is back with the weight loaded on the ball of the back foot. Arms are bent at the elbows and the spine is upright and extended. Lower the back knee in a straight line under the hip toward the floor (see figure *a*). Try to get the front thigh parallel to the floor. With power, lift the front foot and leg upward quickly (see figure *b*). Think about driving the knee straight up toward the ceiling. Maintain the flexion in the back knee. Avoid leaning back as you drive the front knee up, and stay on the ball of the back foot during the entire exercise.

Pendulum Lunge

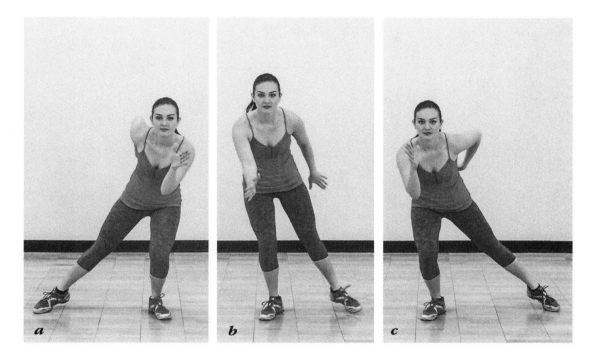

Begin with the feet much wider than hip-width apart and the weight on the left foot, with the right toe just touching the floor. From an upright posture, shift your weight quickly from foot to foot, alternating the weight distribution from foot to toe, but maintain the upright spine (see figures *a-c*). As you shift your weight from side to side, think about pulling your leg in while the other leg reaches out. Continue to shift your weight from foot to toe as you alternate feet, thinking about placing more of the body weight in one leg at a time.

OTHER HIIT EXERCISES

Several other exercises for the lower body are effective for HIIT formats. The squats and lunges just described can be combined with each other and with other movements. These compound sequences require coordinated joint actions and great efforts, which is why they may be appropriate for HIIT formats.

▶ Burpee With Vertical Jump

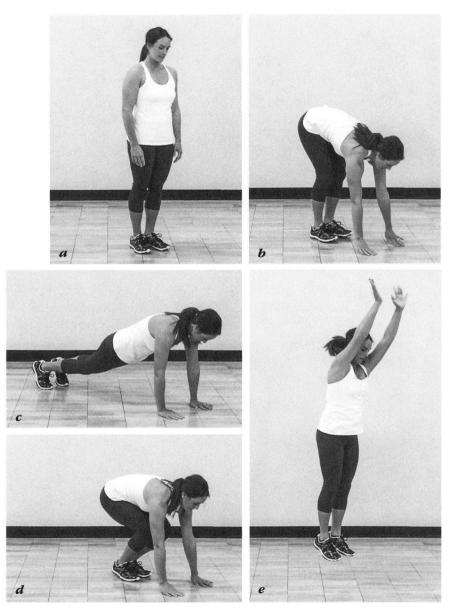

Burpee is another name for squat thrust. To perform a burpee with a vertical jump, begin in a standing position with your feet hip-width apart or closer (see figure *a*); lower your hands to the floor, placing your fingertips on either side of your feet (see figure *b*). Jump back to a push-up position, holding your body in a plank (see figure *c*), and then immediately jump your feet back in toward your hands (see figure *d*) and return to a standing position, immediately jumping straight up with arms reaching straight over your head (see figure *e*).

Burpee With Push-Up

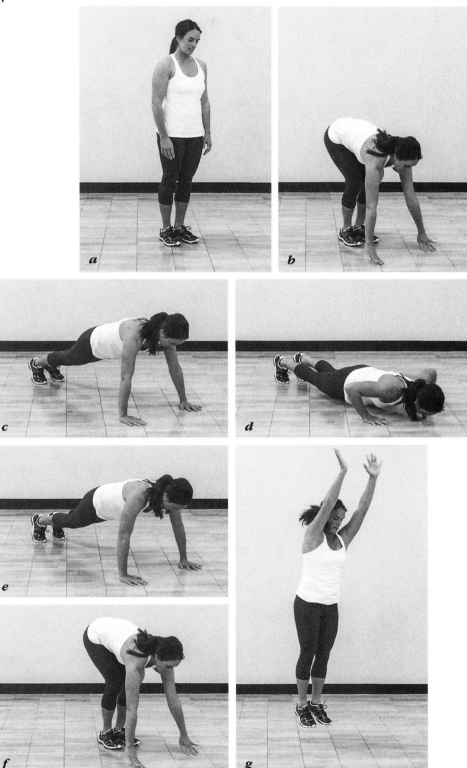

Begin by standing upright (see figure *a*). Lower your hands to the floor while flexing your knees (see figure *b*), and jump back with feet together into a plank position (see figure *c*). Maintain strong, extended, straight arms and a solid, braced core as you lower and come back up performing a push-up (see figures *d* and *e*). Immediately jump your feet back (see figure *f*), and return to a standing position, immediately jumping straight up with arms reaching straight over your head (see figure *g*).

▶ Mountain Climber

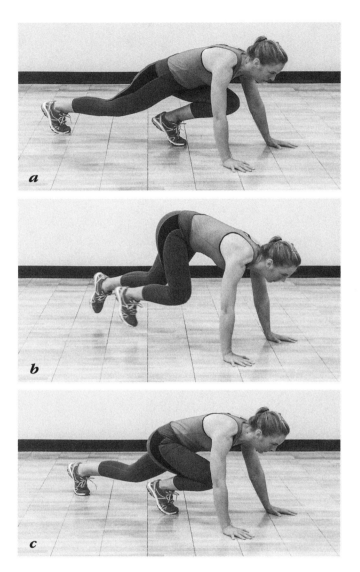

Begin in plank pose with hands slightly in front of the shoulders, fingers spread, and shoulder blades pulled back and down. Hinge the hips up slightly, bringing the left foot forward, and place it slightly under the chest (see figure *a*). The left hip is flexed, and the left knee is pulled in close to the chest while the right leg is extended, supporting the body on the ball of the right foot. Jump to switch feet (see figure *b*), pulling the right knee into the chest while the left leg goes out long and strong (see figure *c*). Continue to alternate legs as you jump or step the feet in and out.

Dolphin Push-Up

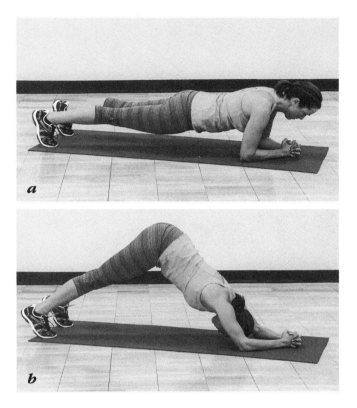

Begin in forearm plank (see figure *a*), clasping the hands together under the center of the chest and allowing the elbows to angle outside the frame of the body. Keeping the toes in contact with the floor and maintaining the plank, pike the hips up toward the ceiling, maintaining a hinge in the hips with an extended spine and straight legs (see figure *b*). Lower back down to plank and repeat.

▶ Speedskater

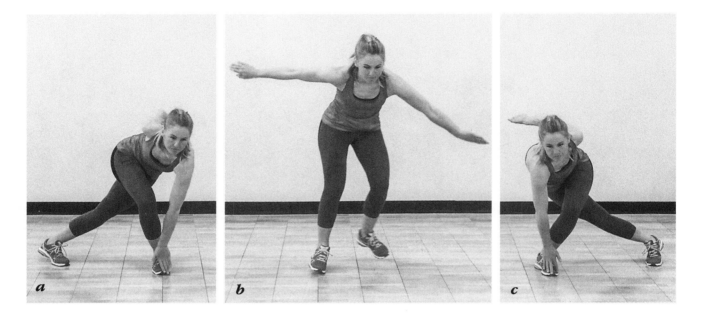

Begin by standing with your feet side by side. Step back with the left leg, flexing the knee and placing the ball of the left foot slightly back, loading weight onto that foot. Lower into an athletic stance, reaching the left hand down until it is directly on top of the right foot (see figure *a*). The spine is extended and the hip is hinged. Alternate legs behind you, reaching out and touching the floor with each pass (see figures *b* and *c*). Allow the back leg to drive through the hip. Stay low and move quickly and smoothly with power.

Mogul Twist

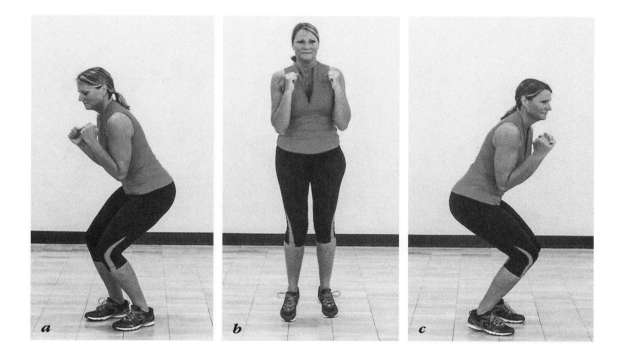

Begin from a standing position, feet close together, hips flexed, and core braced. Imagine standing on a clock face with both feet pointing at 12 o'clock. Lower your center of gravity and jump with both feet to the left (see figure *a*), landing at 3 o'clock and then back over to 9 o'clock (see figures *b* and *c*).

Twist

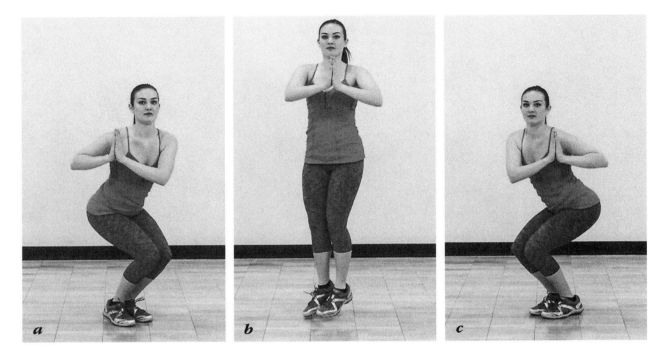

Begin by standing tall with the spine extended and feet as close to each other as possible. Clasp your hands together in front of your chest in a prayer position, pulling the shoulder blades down and pointing the elbows slightly down and out. Begin to twist by pointing the toes from the right to the left. The feet turn one way, and the hands and arms of the upper body pull across the midline of the body in the opposite direction (see figures *a-c*). Try to maintain tension in the muscles of the back and the scapulae by keeping the hands and arms engaged during the entire movement.

Power Speed Skip

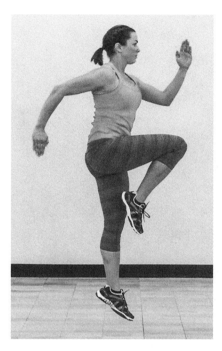

From a standing position, drive the right knee straight up while simultaneously hopping off the left foot (see figure). Use the arms to drive the movement, and power your body straight up in a jump. Continue alternating the knee drive and the hop.

Jumping Jack With Arms to Front

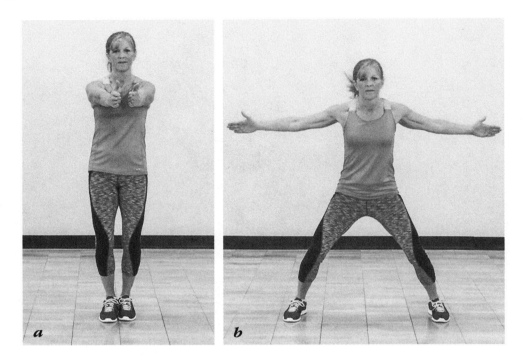

Begin with feet together and arms extended directly in front of the chest (see figure *a*). As you jump out into a jack, open the arms out wide to shoulder height with elbows fully extended (see figure *b*). Return to the starting position and repeat.

HIIT AND PLYOMETRICS

Power moves and jumps called plyometrics are common in HIIT workouts and are often the focus of lower-body exercises. These exercises are usually referenced as those that cause oxygen debt in working muscles and "the burn" in the lungs. Plyometric exercises are beneficial for HIIT workouts because they can help create appropriate overload for the body through increased power output in both the upper body and lower body, target specific muscles, increase muscular endurance and strength, increase mobility, add challenge, and assist the body in crossing the anaerobic threshold. Plyometric exercises that are often part of HIIT workouts are the squat jump, lunges, hops, sprints, and power push-ups. Any exercise that is explosive and includes a quick, power-producing jump, hop, or leap is considered to be in the category of plyometrics.

The purpose of plyometrics in HIIT is to create physical overload. This occurs because plyometrics captures the energy produced immediately after a muscle is lengthened (an eccentric contraction), which commonly precedes concentric muscle actions, or muscle shortening, in powerful sport movements such as jumping and sprinting.

To understand the purpose of plyometric exercises in HIIT workouts, it is important to understand how plyometrics works. Muscles function like springs, absorbing energy and then releasing it, which is also known as the stretch–shortening cycle. This cycle harnesses nervous impulses that travel though the muscles. In milliseconds, a neural message is sent from the lengthened muscles to the spinal cord, which signals the muscles to initiate a powerful contraction. The muscles are rapidly stretched under a load (e.g., gravity) and are in the amortization phase, a sequence in the stretch–shortening cycle in which working muscles are absorbing energy. If the amortization phase lasts too long, the absorbed energy is lost as heat. If it is timed just right, the harnessed energy allows for huge, powerful muscle contractions. Faster movements can often result in stronger contractions, and with plyometric training, force production can be increased as more muscle fibers are used for work. This results in increased caloric expenditure and greater excess postexercise oxygen consumption (EPOC). However, with plyometric exercises comes an increased potential for overuse injuries and burnout. For these reasons, plyometric exercises should be incorporated into workouts only during two or three nonconsecutive days per week.

The lower-body exercise library offers several options for your HIIT workouts. Most of the exercises presented here can be regressed (made easier or more manageable) or progressed (made more challenging) to meet your needs. Harnessing the power of plyometric exercises can also be a key in the development of in-workout fatigue, and will be the foundation of your HIIT program. In the following chapters, you will learn upper-body and core exercises and how to progress and regress them. Once you have an understanding of the exercises, you will be ready to develop workouts to create explosive and effective HIIT programs to attain the best training results possible.

6

UPPER-BODY EXERCISES

Training the upper body is critical for muscular strength and overall core stability. Plus, upper-body training is important to include in your HIIT workouts because it will assist you in balancing your workouts biomechanically. The muscles of the upper body are numerous and complex and important to develop for total-body strength and function.

When performing the upper-body exercises, you will notice a more pronounced local muscle fatigue, as opposed to the overall fatigue that causes breathlessness during HIIT lower-body exercises. Because muscles adapt to stress quickly, typically adjusting to a particular exercise in only six to eight workouts, you will need to perform a variety of upper-body exercises to maintain a state of progressive overload. This is why there are several exercises for each muscle group, as well as variations using body weight, tubing, and dumbbells. This variety will help you achieve the overload and therefore the training results you are looking for.

This chapter guides you through a variety of the best upper-body exercises to include in your HIIT workouts and explains what they are most beneficial for and how to perform them for optimal results. You will learn the major muscles of the upper body, where they are located, and what they do to assist you in day-to-day, real-life activities.

UPPER-BODY MUSCLES

Because the upper-body muscles work so closely together, they should be trained as a group, focusing on training the movements. You will also want to adopt a functional approach to their training, considering how they work and what they do for your body in everyday life. The major muscles of the upper body are those of the back, chest, shoulders, and arms.

Back Muscles

The major muscles of the back are the latissimus dorsi, trapezius, rhomboids, and spinal erectors. These muscles allow for shoulder adduction and abduction, internal and external rotation, elevation of the scapulae, and extension, and flexion of the neck and low back. These muscles allow you to move the upper body freely, with power and strength. See figure 6.1 for an illustration of the upper-body back muscles.

The latissimus dorsi, the largest of the upper-body muscles, are fan-shaped muscles along the sides of the body. They start low on the spine, spread across the width of the back, and taper off where the upper arm meets the shoulder joint. Building your

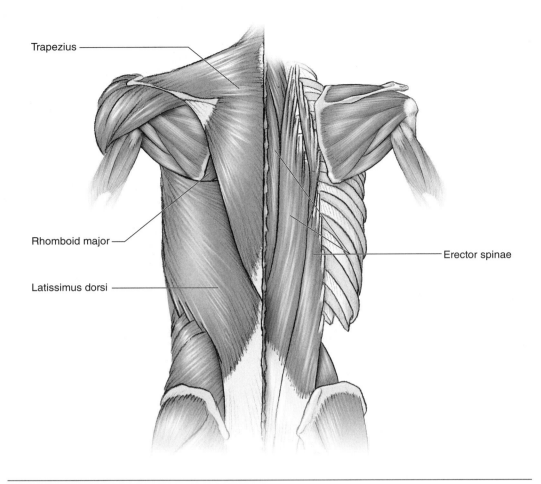

Trapezius

Rhomboid major

Latissimus dorsi

Erector spinae

Figure 6.1 The back muscles.

lats (as they are commonly called) can give your back a wider, flared appearance that tapers down to your waist in a V shape that creates the illusion of a smaller waistline. These large posterior muscles assist the body in performing most pulling motions, as well as reaching the arms out and away from the body and then bringing them back into the sides again. Several exercises for the latissimus dorsi are useful for creating strength, emphasizing definition, improving posture, and enhancing core stability.

The trapezius is a flat, triangular muscle that begins at the base of the skull or the top of the neck and inserts itself at the back of the collarbone and shoulder blades, offering a desirable muscular shape to the upper part of the back and shoulders. The trapezius helps to draw the shoulder blades together and down, as well as to shrug the arms and shoulders up.

The rhomboids, which work closely with the trapezius, are diamond-shaped muscles that lie in the middle of the upper back between the shoulder blades and directly underneath the trapezius. The rhomboids assist the trapezius in pulling the shoulders blades together, which can help in any activity that requires pulling.

Last, the spinal erectors are often also called the low back muscles, but they actually begin at the base of the skull and taper all the way down the back. They are composed of two columns of muscles, one on each side of the spine. The spinal erectors straighten the spine after spinal flexion, as well as allow for spinal extension (straight, proper posture) or arching the back, so they are very important for core strength, stability, and proper, upright posture.

Chest Muscles

The muscles on the front of the upper body are the chest muscles. The pectoralis major is a fan-shaped muscle that starts at the center of the breastbone and stretches wide across each side of the chest, finally connecting at the upper arm bone (the humerus). The pectoralis minor lies beneath it. A thinner muscle, it starts at the ribs and also connects at the upper arm. The chest muscles have the job of moving the arms inward and across the midline of the body at various angles. These muscles also work with the arms and shoulders to perform pushing movements such as pushing a shopping cart or a stroller or performing a plank or push-up. See figure 6.2 for an illustration of the upper-body chest muscles.

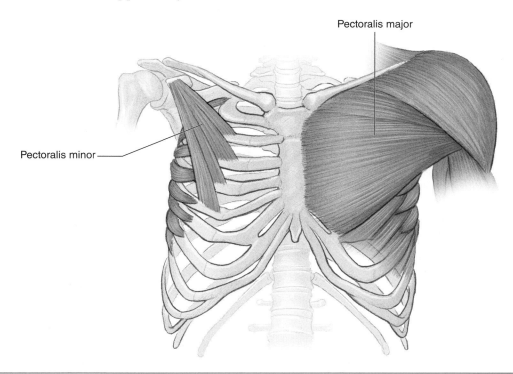

Figure 6.2 The chest muscles.

Shoulder Muscles

The shoulders are composed of the three separate deltoid muscles—the anterior, medial, and posterior heads—and the four rotator cuff muscles that hold the upper arm into the shoulder joint. The deltoid group consists of the anterior (front) and medial (middle or top) deltoids, located on the front and top of the shoulder; they begin on the collarbone. The posterior deltoids are located on the back of the shoulder joints and attach to the scapulae (shoulder blades). The deltoids play a large role in extending the arms in all directions. The anterior deltoids lift the arms up in front of the body. The medial deltoids raise the arms out to the sides, and the posterior deltoids lift the arms up behind—for example, when drawing the elbows together or reaching back. The deltoids also assist the rotator cuff muscles in rotating the shoulders both internally and externally. Strong, balanced deltoids help decrease the risk of shoulder joint injury. See figure 6.3 for an illustration of the shoulder muscles.

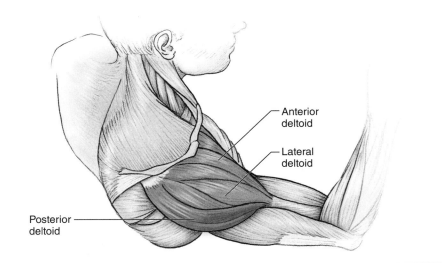

Figure 6.3 The shoulder muscles.

The rotator cuff is made up of four shoestring-like muscles, often called the SITS muscle, an acronym for the muscles' proper names: supraspinatus, infraspinatus, and teres minor. The rotator cuff is responsible for stabilizing the shoulder joint and for rotational movements in all directions. The rotator cuff works with the other, more superficial muscles of the shoulder to stabilize the joint. The shoulder is unique in that it is very mobile, but as a result it is also very unstable, predisposing it to injury. Therefore, care must be taken when performing movements involving the shoulder joints. We work very hard to protect the shoulder joint in all the HIIT exercises described in these workouts. However, the more awareness you have regarding shoulder movements, the more stable these joints will be and the lower your risk for shoulder injury will be. See figure 6.4 for an illustration of the rotator cuff muscles.

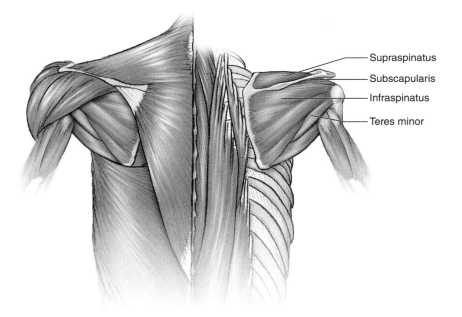

Figure 6.4 The rotator cuff muscles.

Arm Muscles

The muscles of the arms include the biceps and triceps. The biceps is located on the front of the upper arm above the elbow and on the lower arm just below the elbow, running into the forearms. It is responsible for elbow flexion and contributes to wrist stability and grip strength. The biceps flexes the elbow, bringing the hands closer to the shoulders. It also supinates the wrist, which turns the palms faceup (supine) or down (prone) in rotation and sets the hand in a neutral position (thumb pointed up). The biceps also assists with shoulder flexion.

The arm muscle on the back of the upper arm is the triceps. The triceps is made up of three muscles: the lateral, medial, and long heads. The lateral and medial heads both start on the upper arm bone (the humerus), whereas the long head starts at the shoulder blade. All three come together and attach to an insertion point on a bone at the elbow joint called the ulna. The main job of the triceps is to straighten the arms by extending the elbow. It is also used in conjunction with the chest muscles during pressing movements or chest exercises such as the chest press, push-up, and plank. See figure 6.5 for an illustration of the arm muscles.

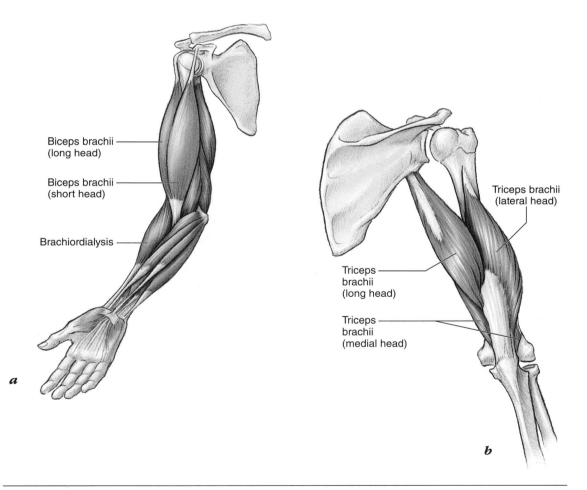

Figure 6.5 The arm muscles: *(a)* anterior view and *(b)* posterior view.

FOUNDATIONAL MOVEMENTS FOR THE UPPER BODY

Foundational movements are standardized body-weight exercises moving specific joint ranges of motion in particular planes of motion. For example, a plank is a foundational move for the upper body and core that is performed in the sagittal plane. To execute the plank correctly and safely, you need to understand its purpose, which muscles should feel tension, and what a correct plank looks and feels like.

Following are descriptions of foundational upper-body exercises that can be used in HIIT workouts, including how to execute them at the most basic level as well as additional options. Chapter 8 describes many exercise sequence options.

Foundational Movement 1: Plank

The plank is an important isometric exercise that that can be very powerful in the assessment of upper-body and core strength, posture, and spinal stability. When performed properly, the plank can enhance endurance, power, and strength in the back, chest, arms, and torso. A full plank (performed from the hands as opposed to the forearms) can even increase the stability of the wrists, elbows, and shoulder girdle, contributing to an improved awareness of spinal length.

The plank is a foundational movement for all facedown (prone) hand- or forearm-stabilized moves in addition to almost any exercise in which the body is in an extended spinal position. A proper upright standing posture as well as a lunge could even be viewed as a plank, because no matter what the position of the body, you are looking for upright posture with the shoulder, hip, outside of the knee, and ankle aligned. Chapter 8 presents exercise options that combine several body postures, such as a burpee, a lunge, and a two-knee push-up; in all of these, the plank is a performance factor. For example, when you are down on both knees performing a push-up, you must be aware of the plank pose (ear, shoulder, hip, and knee) to ensure proper spinal alignment. Even though both hands and all of your toes are not on the floor, it is a still a plank pose. This is why you must always heed the plank guidelines when performing any movements for which proper posture, particularly spinal extension, is key. In all of the exercises in this chapter, the plank posture is integral to proper movement execution.

Practicing the plank can improve strength in the back and neck and help develop a stronger abdominal area when in upright postures because it involves an isometric muscular contraction that mimics upright stances. Even though the plank is often considered a core exercise (which it is), it is a very powerful movement for upper-body training, too. It is often assumed that the plank can be performed well without instruction, but it is important to understand how to set up a proper plank to gain all the benefits and decrease the risk of injury.

Basic Full Plank

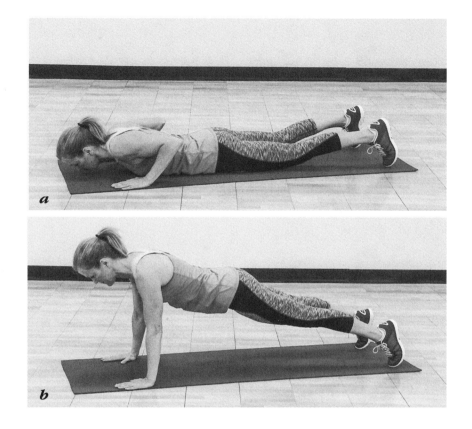

Begin by lying facedown with your body straight. Place your feet hip-width apart with the toes dug into the floor, the hands directly under the shoulders, the fingers spread, and the index fingers pointing forward with the elbows pointing up and behind, like a grasshopper's legs (see figure *a*). Press the heels toward the wall behind you using the toes and forefeet to create leverage. Contract the quads, lifting the kneecaps up through the thigh muscles, and tighten the abdominal muscles. Prepare by taking a deep breath in and then exhale as you press straight up, as if pushing into the top phase of a push-up (see figure *b*). This is the plank position. In plank position, you should be able to draw an imaginary plumb line from your ear, straight down through your shoulder, to the side of your hip and knee, and all the way to the outside ankle bone. If this line is straight, your body is likely in correct plank pose.

Refine your plank position by checking to see that your hands are under your shoulders with your shoulder blades pulled down, neck elongated, and chin tucked slightly as the crown of your head extends forward. Draw an imaginary line between your thumbs and place your sternum (breastbone) directly over the line. This will cause you to shift your body weight slightly forward, placing more stress on the chest, shoulders, hands, and arms.

Basic Push-Up

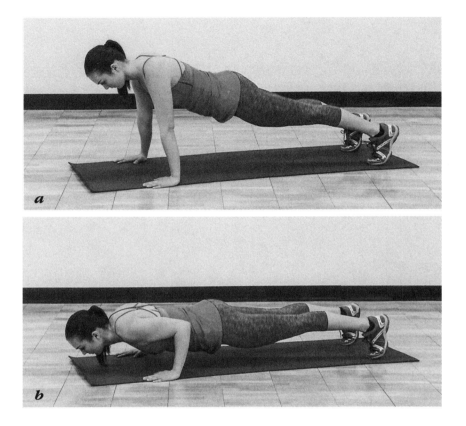

Begin by placing your hands flat on the floor with the arms straight and elbows slightly bent, as in plank position (see figure *a*). Your legs will be straight behind you with your feet either hip-width apart or slightly together. Rise up onto your toes so the tops of the balls of your feet are touching the floor. Your body should be in one straight line—from the top of your head to your heels. Your eyes should be focused straight down at the floor, and the crown of your head should be extended forward. Without lowering your head, lower yourself until your upper arms are parallel to the floor (see figure *b*). Pause, slowly push yourself back up, and repeat. This can be done with one or both knees down.

Triceps Push-Up

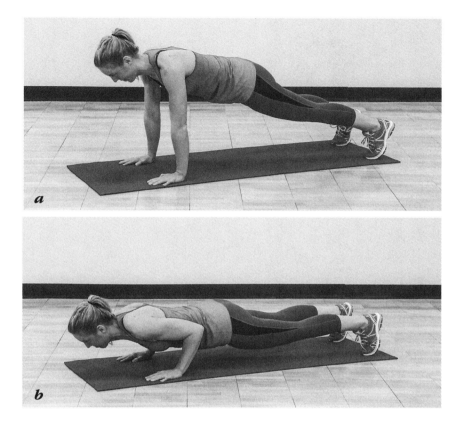

Begin by placing your hands flat on the floor with the arms straight and elbows slightly bent, as in plank position with the hands directly under the shoulders, fingers spread (see figure *a*). Your legs will be straight behind you with your feet either hip-width apart or slightly together. Rise up onto your toes so the balls of your feet are touching the floor. Your body should be in one straight line—from the crown of your head to your heels. Your eyes should be focused straight down to the floor. Without lowering your head, lower yourself until your upper arms are parallel to the floor and aligned directly by your sides (see figure *b*). Pause, slowly push yourself back up, and repeat. As you perform the triceps push-up, keep the arms close to the sides of the body. You can make this exercise more manageable by placing one knee or both knees on the floor.

Military-Style Push-Up

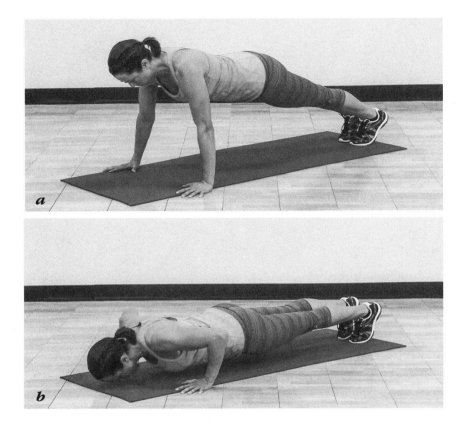

Begin by placing your hands flat on the floor with the arms straight and elbows just slightly bent, as in plank position with the hands directly under the shoulders but wider than shoulder width (see figure *a*). The fingers should be spread, and the elbows should create a 90-degree angle at the bottom of the push-up and straighten at the top. Without lowering your head, lower yourself until your upper arms are parallel to the floor (see figure *b*). Pause, slowly push yourself back up, and repeat.

Two-Knee Push-Up

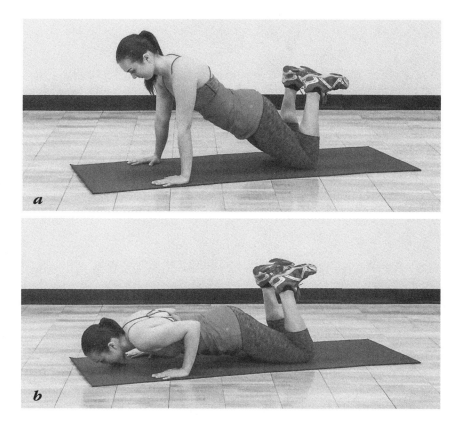

Lie facedown placing the hands directly under the shoulders with fingers spread and elbows facing back. Bend your knees by pulling your feet closer to your hips, and push yourself up into the plank position (see figure *a*). Lower your body until your elbows flex and you are as low as you can be while remaining stable (see figure *b*). Pause, and then slowly press yourself back up and repeat.

▶ One-Knee Push-Up

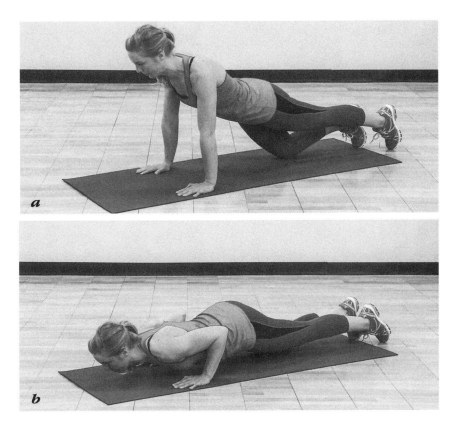

Face down, placing the hands directly under the shoulders with fingers spread and elbows facing back as in a plank position. The body will be at approximately a 45-degree angle (see figure *a*). Placing one knee on the floor as you lower into the bottom of the range of motion of the push up, lower yourself until your elbows flex maximally (see figure *b*). Alternating which knee you lower will create balance in the exercise.

Foundational Movement 2: Pulling and Pressing

Being able to push and press properly will assist you in everyday activities. You can see by all the plank and push-ups we just examined, proper plank alignment, is key to proper execution and performance of any pressing movement, including standing movements using resistance tubing. Pulling is also important in activities of daily living, assists us with the ability to bring objects closer to us, and helps us perform exercises properly. Proper pulling technique will yield great results in the ability to lift, climb, and run as well as improve muscular balance and posture. The plank alignment is also an important component of performing the pulling movements correctly.

The following exercises incorporate either pulling or pressing movements using tools such as tubing, dumbbells, a medicine ball, or a kettlebell. Equipment is necessary for achieving the overload you need to make these upper-body exercises effective.

Chest Press

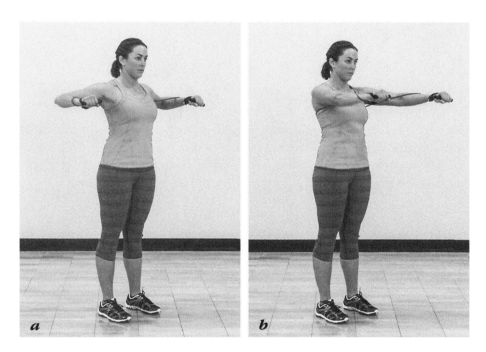

Use your body as an anchor and wrap resistance tubing around your back so that the handles come out from under your armpits (see figure *a*). With the palms facing down, press the handles out, directly in front of the shoulders, until the elbows are fully extended (see figure *b*). Pause and then return by flexing the elbows and bringing the hands back to the shoulders.

Single-Arm Press

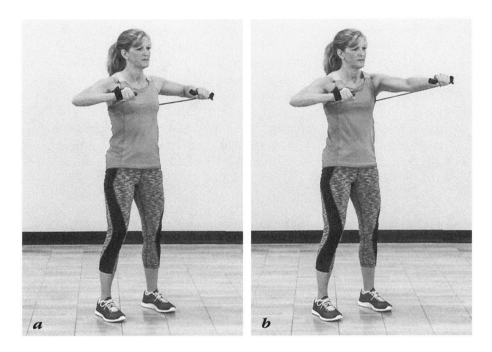

Use your body as an anchor and wrap long tubing around your back so that the handles come out from under your armpits (see figure *a*). With the palms facing down, press one arm out directly in front of the shoulders until the elbow is fully extended (see figure *b*). Repeat with the other arm.

Chest Fly

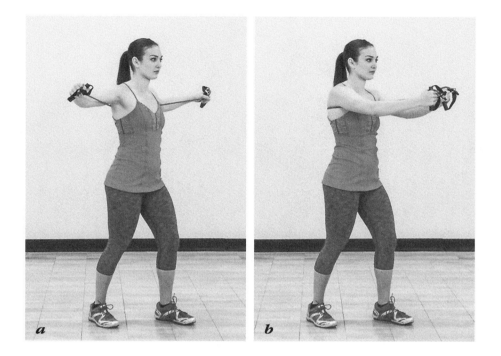

Use your body as an anchor and wrap long tubing around your back so that the handles come out from under your armpits. Spread your arms wide (see figure *a*). With the palms facing each other, press out and then cross the midline of the body, bringing the hands together in a slight arc in front of the chest (see figure *b*); then return to the bent-arm position.

Lat Pulldown

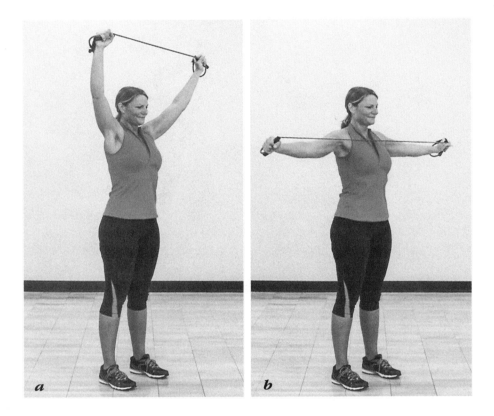

Using a resistance tube, grasp the handles and shorten the tubing by wrapping it around your hands or wrists to create the correct line of pull. Hold the tubing above your head but slightly in front of your body, with your arms pulled apart and your elbows straight (see figure *a*). Keep tension in the tubing with your head upright and your spine extended; pull the tubing down in front of your body until it reaches your chest. Hold the tubing at your chest for a short pause (see figure *b*), and then raise the hands back up above your head with your elbows extended.

Single-Arm Pulldown

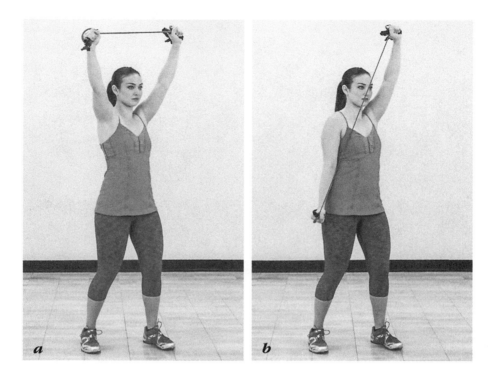

Using a resistance tube, grasp the handles and shorten the tubing by wrapping it around your hands or wrists to create the correct line of pull. Hold the tubing above your head but slightly in front of your body, with your arms pulled slightly apart and your elbows straight (see figure *a*). Keep your head upright and your spine extended, pulling the tubing down using one arm at a time (see figure *b*). Hold the tubing at the bottom of the movement for a short pause, and then raise your arm back up above your head with your elbow extended and repeat with the other arm.

▶ **Bent-Over Row**

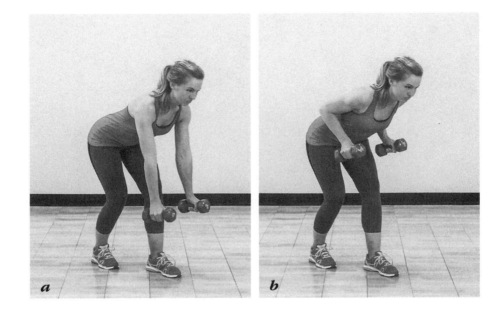

Stand with feet in a lunge stance with one foot in front of the other, knees slightly bent. Lean forward in a hinge with the spine extended, holding a dumbbell in each hand (see figure *a*). The arms should be hanging straight down with the palms facing each other. Keeping your arms close to your torso, raise both dumbbells up until they reach the sides of your chest (see figure *b*). The elbows should point straight up behind your body. Pause at the top and slowly lower the dumbbells until your arms are straight once more.

Single-Arm Bent-Over Row

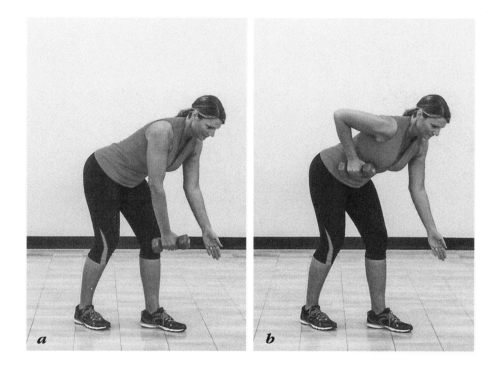

Stand with feet in a lunge stance with one foot in front of the other, knees slightly bent. Lean forward in a hinge with the spine extended, holding a dumbbell in one hand (see figure *a*). The arms should be hanging straight down with the palms facing each other. Keeping your arm close to your torso, raise the dumbbell until it reaches the side of your chest (see figure *b*). The elbow should point straight up behind your body. Pause at the top and slowly lower the dumbbell until your arm is straight once more.

Seated Row

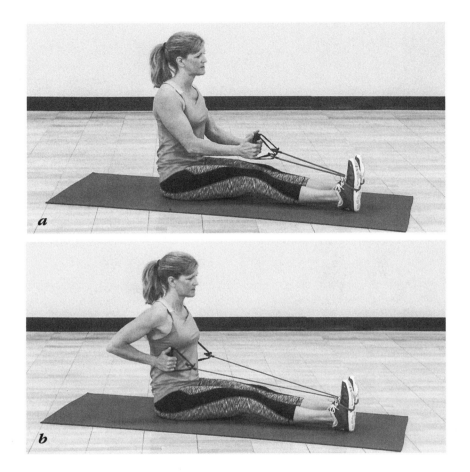

Sit with your back against a wall or in a very upright posture, and bend your knees as much as necessary to extend your spine fully. With both arms extended and resistance tubing wrapped around the bottoms of both feet securely, grasp a handle in each hand with the palms facing each other (see figure *a*). Pull your hands toward your torso, squeezing your back by drawing your shoulder blades together while maintaining an upright posture until the arms are near the rib cage (see figure *b*). Pause and return to the starting position.

Shoulder Press

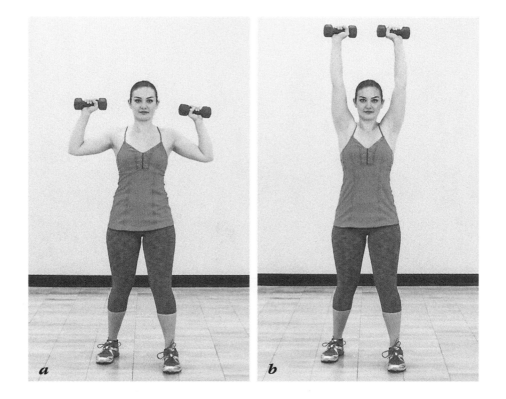

Stand with your feet shoulder-width apart (or wider if you need more stability), and hold a dumbbell in each hand. Bring the dumbbells to just above your shoulders by your ears with your elbows pointing down and your palms facing forward (see figure *a*). Slowly press the dumbbells up and over your head with your hands slightly in front of your head (see figure *b*). Keep your spine erect and extended as you press up. Lower the dumbbells to your shoulders.

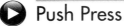 Push Press

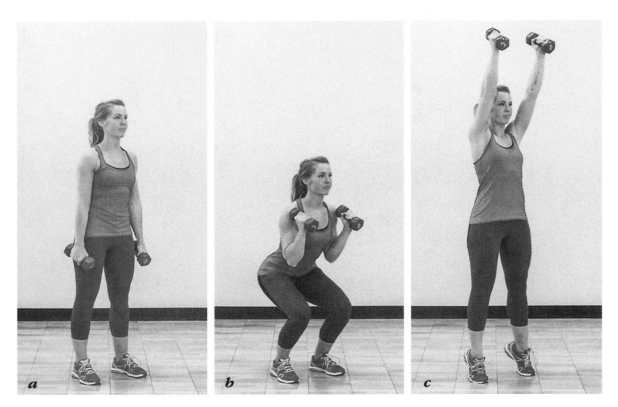

Stand holding a dumbbell in each hand (see figure *a*). Flex your elbows, pointing them down to the floor and forearms parallel to the floor. Squat and continue to hold the elbows close to the body (see figure *b*); then quickly rise up on the toes, simultaneously pressing the arms up and over your head (see figure *c*). Lower the dumbbells to your shoulders and repeat from the squat. Keep your forearms close to the sides of your body.

Upright Row With Dumbbells

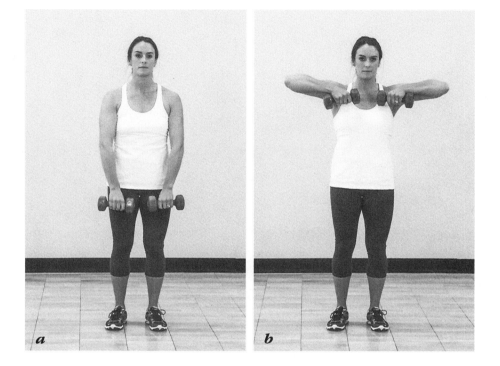

Stand tall with feet shoulder-width apart and a dumbbell in each hand. Allow your arms to hang in front of your body so that the dumbbells rest on your upper thighs, palms facing your body (see figure *a*). Slowly draw the dumbbells up toward your chin allowing the elbows to point out to the sides (see figure *b*). Lift your hands only to shoulder height, and try to keep your wrists and elbows at the same height. Pause at the top and focus on keeping the neck extended and the shoulders down away from the ears; then lower to the starting position.

Upright Row With Tubing

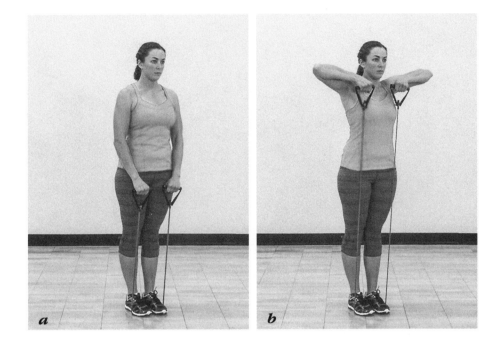

Place long resistance tubing under both feet. Be sure the tubing is secure and grasp the handles in each hand. Hold your hands in front of and facing your body, maintaining tension in the tubing (see figure *a*). Draw the hands up toward your shoulders, allowing the elbows to drive up and out to the sides of the body, and bring the handles to shoulder height (see figure *b*). Maintain an extended neck and keep your chin level with the floor. Pause at the top, and slowly release back down to the starting position.

Lateral Raise With Dumbbells

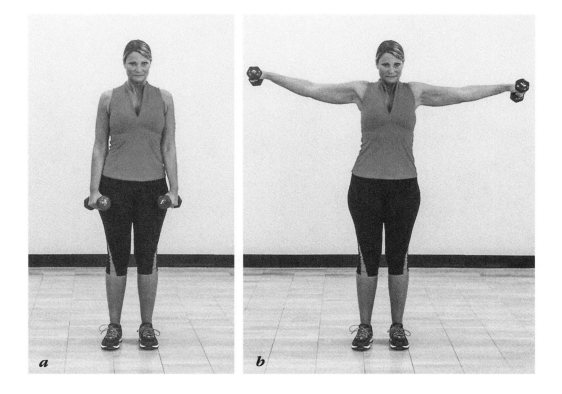

Standing with your feet hip-width apart, hold a dumbbell in each hand. Your hands should hang down at your sides, and your palms should face each other (see figure *a*). Keeping your arms straight, slowly raise them out and up toward your shoulders until your arms are parallel to the floor and look like the letter T (see figure *b*). Pause at the top of the movement, and then, with control, lower the dumbbells to your sides.

▶ Lateral Raise With Tubing

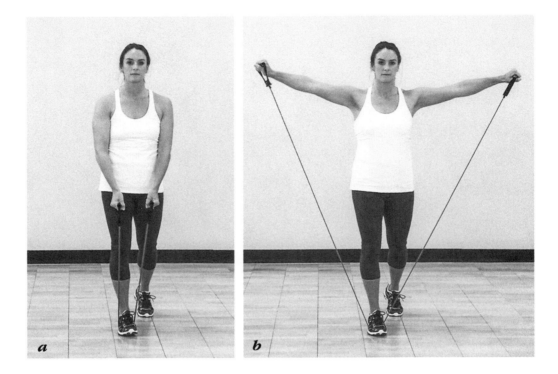

Stand in a staggered stance with the right foot in front of the left, and anchor the tubing under your right foot; the resistance should be evenly distributed between your hands (see figure *a*). Your arms should hang down by your sides slightly in front of your body with the palms facing each other. Under control, raise the palms up and out to the sides until they are at shoulder height (see figure *b*). Pause at the top of the movement, and then, with control, lower your hands to your sides.

Biceps Curl

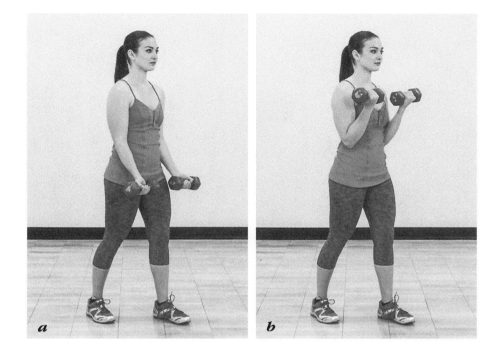

Stand with a dumbbell in each hand and your arms hanging at your sides; your palms should be facing forward (see figure *a*). Keep your spine extended, and slowly curl the dumbbells up toward your shoulders (see figure *b*). Your palms should end up facing the fronts of your shoulders. Slowly lower the dumbbells. This exercise can be done with tubing, a kettlebell, or any load you can hold in your hand or palm.

Single-Arm Biceps Curl

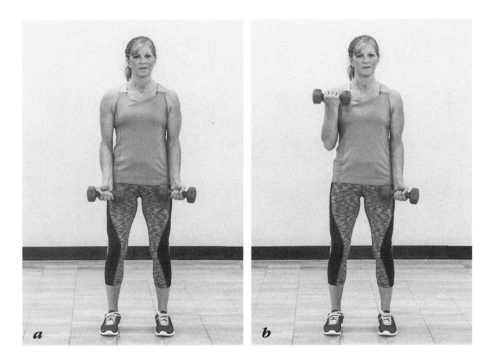

Stand with a dumbbell in each hand and your arms hanging at your sides; your palms should be facing forward (see figure *a*). Keep your spine extended, and slowly curl one arm up toward your shoulder (see figure *b*). Your palm should end up facing the front of your shoulder. Slowly lower the dumbbell, and repeat with the other arm. This exercise can be done using tubing, a kettlebell, or any load you can hold in your hand or palm.

Triceps Kickback

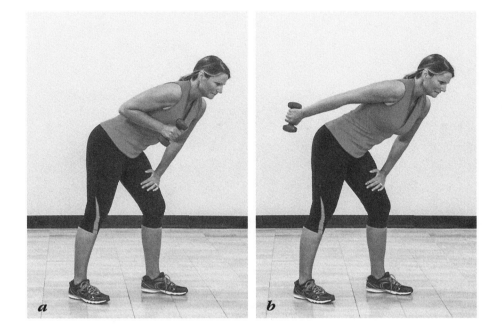

Stand with your feet in a staggered stance (left leg in front and right leg in back) with a dumbbell in your right hand. The toes of the front foot point forward, and the toes of the back foot turn out about 45 degrees. Lightly lean onto your left thigh with your left hand as you flex your right elbow and bring the dumbbell toward the shoulder (see figure *a*). Extend the right elbow back, pushing the weight behind you until the elbow joint is fully extended (see figure *b*). Pause and then return to the starting position. After a specific time frame, switch arms and legs and perform the exercise for the same time frame on the other side.

▶ Quadruped Triceps Press

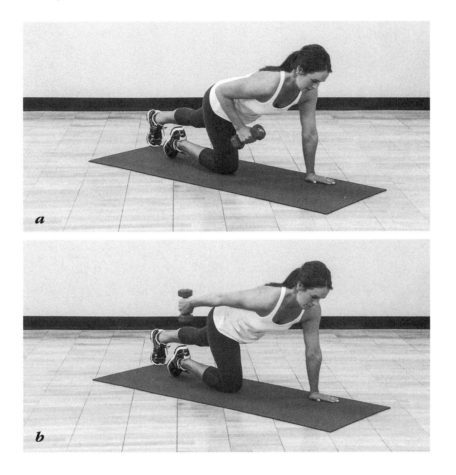

From an all-fours position (on hands and knees), extend your left leg behind you, securing the foot by digging the toes into the floor. Try to maintain a long, strong body as you align yourself. Hold a dumbbell in your right hand close to your shoulder with your elbow flexed and aligned with the side of your body (see figure *a*). Extend the right elbow, raising the weight behind your body so the arm is fully extended, but keeping the upper arm close to the side of the body (see figure *b*). Pause and then return to the starting position. For more challenge, extend the left leg up, so the foot is at hip height, using the gluteal muscles to hold the leg in place. Switch arms as indicated by the timing technique.

Although the exercises listed here are relatively basic, the variations, as well as the time frames, recovery between exercises, and combinations presented in chapter 8, 9, and 10, will keep your body challenged but balanced. Mastering the basics and then adding the new exercises will bring increased overload and even better training results. When the lower-body, upper-body, and core exercises are combined (in chapter 8), these moves provide total-body exercise routines and recipes for perfect results to help you avoid exercise plateaus.

Starting with large muscle groups and moving to smaller ones is best. For example, many of the upper-body intervals start with the back and chest and move to the biceps and triceps. If you fatigue the small muscles too quickly, they will not be able to do their job as well (which is to stabilize the joints that are used when larger muscles are active). This may cause premature fatigue and an inability to exhaust the larger muscles, which will not bring about desired fitness improvements.

Chapter 7 concludes the exercise chapters by offering some of the most effective body-weight and equipment-based core exercises available. Once you can incorporate lower-body, upper-body, and core exercises into your HIIT routines, you will begin to see the results you are looking for.

CORE EXERCISES

This chapter takes you through the final collection of HIIT exercises, focusing primarily on the important and powerful muscles of the core. The term *core training* is frequently considered synonymous with *abdominal training* and is often referenced when someone has abdominal muscles that are lean, cut, and defined, which is known as having a great six-pack. However, there is significantly more to core training than just training the abdominals. Additionally, some people make efforts to train the core by using a variety of complicated balance movements on an assortment of fitness equipment. The truth is that core training is so much more than just six-pack abdominal training or balance training. The core muscles do include the abdominal muscles, and balance can be traced back to good core control, but the muscles of the core also include the gluteals and the front and back of the torso.

Consider the muscles of the core beginning at the collar bone and running all the way through the middle of the thigh. In fact, every muscle that passes through the pelvis and all the muscles that attach to the spinal column are considered the core—more than 30 in all. And because the core muscles are attached to the legs, shoulders, and arms, the core carries the burden of supporting the entire body. If the muscles of the core are not well developed and strong and able to work comprehensively with other muscles and joints, the entire burden of supporting the body would be on the bones, joints, and skin. So you can see that the core is necessary to support your body weight during any type of movement, including standing, sitting, walking, running, and all types of exercise.

A LITTLE MORE ABOUT THE CORE

The core refers to your center of gravity, which is most commonly just below the belly button. The muscle structure of the core operates most effectively in upright standing, walking, and running postures. The core muscles respond to the pull of gravity on the body, as well as ground reaction forces, as they attempt to stabilize the torso (including the thoracic spine and rib cage), which is moving in opposition to the pelvis, or hips. The core muscles create and develop power in the gluteals and transfer that energy back out through the arms and legs, allowing for functional movement. This is one reason that using crunches to sculpt the abs may be detrimental to functional core training.

This is not to say that crunches are not useful in a HIIT program, but they are only one of a collection of exercises that will create powerful, functional core stability and strength. The main purpose of the core muscles is to limit and control rotational multiplanar movements. During movement, effort should be made to control and

(continued)

┌───┐
A Little More About the Core *(continued)*

stabilize the spine, using the core as a brace or corset. When the core is engaged in this way, it helps to steady and direct the body. Because this takes significant effort, energy, and focus, core training needs to be very specific, precise, and organized.

The fact that upright postures have powerful effects on the core is great news for those performing HIIT training—many of the HIIT exercises in this book are performed upright. So even when you are performing the lower-body exercises that are primarily for creating oxygen debt to take you across the anaerobic threshold (e.g., jumping, squatting, and lunging), as well as many of the upper-body exercises (e.g., the plank and push-up), you are also working the core. The routines in this book all incorporate core exercises to create a total-body HIIT experience.
└───┘

CORE MUSCLES

The major muscles of the core are the transverse abdominis, internal and external obliques, and rectus abdominis on the front of the torso; the spinal erector muscles on the back (included in upper-body training but also part of the core); and the iliopsoas and gluteus maximus, medius, and minimus in the hips. See figure 7.1 for an illustration of the core muscles.

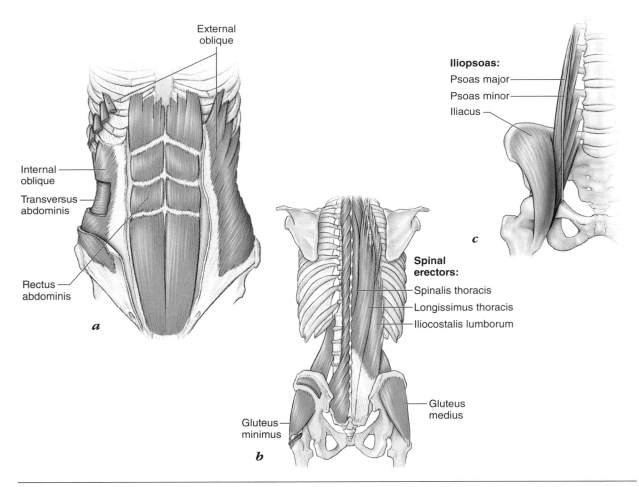

Figure 7.1 The core muscles: *(a)* anterior view and *(b)* posterior view, and *(c)* hips.

Anterior Core Muscles

The transverse abdominis muscle is the deepest of the anterior core and may be considered the most important with respect to core strength. It acts as a corset, holding the contents of the torso in place as well as transferring the strength between the lower and upper body. Also referred to as the TVA, this muscle is not capable of contractions known as isotonic, meaning that it does not actually shorten and lengthen the way, say, a biceps muscle does. Instead, the TVA responds primarily to breathing, performing an isometric (or held) contraction as you exhale. Take a deep breath in and exhale with control as if you were blowing up a balloon. You should feel the engagement of the deep abdominal muscles; these are your TVA muscles contracting as you exhale with control. They are best activated during deep, controlled breathing, which is particularly important during HIIT exercises. Breathing and controlling the breath during these exercises can really enhance the development of this muscle.

The obliques are divided into internal and external (two of each). The internal and external obliques are paired along each side of the waist and lie diagonally across the midsection. These muscles are positioned slightly to the side of the torso and slink all the way up the rib cage. They are responsible for spinal movements including rotation and lateral flexion, or side bending.

The rectus abdominis is the most superficial of the anterior core muscles, lying on top of the other abdominal muscles; this muscle is often called the six-pack. This long muscle begins on the sternum at the center of the rib cage and attaches at the pubic bone. Often described as the upper abs and the lower abs, the rectus abdominis is actually just one long muscle running the length of the front of the torso. The confusion in believing that it is two muscles (upper and lower) comes from the appearance of the tendinous insertions that create the six-pack look. The fact is, when performing

VARIETY IN CORE TRAINING

As mentioned earlier in the book, muscles adapt quickly to stress, typically adjusting to a particular exercise in only six to eight workouts. You should perform a variety of core exercises to help your body maintain a state of progressive overload, as well as continue to perfect the movements and improve strength and stability as part of core training.

Core training, unlike many other types of training, includes subtle movements that you will need to practice over and over to master. This is why there are so many core exercises that look similar. However, slight variations in body positions, particularly in how the body relates to gravity and controls against rotation, make core exercises relatively complex; even simple changes can affect the outcomes. The variety in core training comes from combinations of hand, arm, leg, and foot positions as well as body positions such as back-lying (supine), side-lying, seated, and facedown (prone). These positions require very particular muscular engagement and specific postural control and techniques.

The exercise descriptions in this chapter offer precise details regarding implementation. Keep in mind that the quality of the movement is far more important than the number of repetitions performed. The motto "better is better" could not be more significant when it comes to the core training section of the HIIT workout. To understand core training, we examine the muscles that comprise the core, where they are located, what they do, and how to train them for function, spinal support, better daily and sport performance, and finally, to look great.

exercises in which the rib cage approaches the pelvis, such as a crunch, the top of the rectus abdominis initiates the movement. In exercises in which the pelvis approaches the rib cage (as in the eagle wrap reverse crunch discussed later in this chapter), the bottom of the rectus abdominis initiates the movement. Because of this division of movement, people often perceive the exercise as exclusive to either the upper abs or the lower abs, but actually, the entire abdominal muscle is firing.

Posterior Core Muscles

The spinal erectors, also discussed in chapter 6 as upper-body muscles, are also part of the core. They begin at the base of the skull and taper all the way down the back. Composed of two columns of muscles, one on each side of the spine, the spinal erectors straighten the spine after flexion, or bring it back to upright after bending forward. The spinal erectors also allow for spinal extension, or arching the back, so they are very important for stability and maintaining a proper upright posture.

Hip Muscles

The iliopsoas is also known as the hip flexor and is actually two muscles: the iliacus and the psoas major. They are located at the top of the front of the thighs where the legs attach to the torso. These muscles work in concert with the quadriceps to raise the legs in hip flexion. These muscles join at the top of the leg, travel through the pelvis, and attach onto the low back. Because we tend to do much more sitting than walking or standing, these muscles tend to get tight and pull on the low back, often causing low back pain. The hip flexors need to be lengthened through continuous stretching and strengthening routines to alleviate low back pain and assist with uninhibited movement through the hips and the front of the legs. With greater range of motion, the hip flexors can contribute more to performance outcomes. For example, running with a longer stride and lifting the knees higher with each stride may result in a better running performance and, in the long term, greater caloric expenditure.

The gluteus maximus is one of the largest muscles of the lower body and an important core muscle as well. Although discussed in chapter 5, it is worthy of inclusion in the discussion on core muscles because it plays an important role in the development of core strength. The gluteus maximus is extremely important in any activity that moves the body forward and is critical for the development of good posture, which is essential for a strong core. The gluteus maximus can become weak as a result of improper engagement or too much inactivity (e.g. sitting). It often appears flat and underdeveloped in people whose fitness programs do not capitalize on the multidimensional roles the gluteal muscles play in cardiorespiratory performance, lower-body strength, core strength, and stability.

The gluteus medius and gluteus minimus are both deeper than the more superficial gluteus maximus. The medius is located on the side of the hip area; the minimus is deeper in the hip area. Both are important in the movement of the gluteals as a whole and play a role in outward leg rotation and side lifting as well as side stepping.

CORE TRAINING HEALTH AND SAFETY GUIDELINES

Core exercise selection as part of the prescribed HIIT workouts is addressed in chapters 8 through 10. However, there are a few guidelines you should bear in mind when performing the core exercises as part of your HIIT workouts.

Prioritize Quality Over Quantity

Learning the plank as a foundational move is important so you can perform a quality plank, push-up, or forearm plank every time. In fact, proper plank position is reflective of proper posture for all the exercises described here. If maintaining a quality plank is becoming too difficult, simply take the regression (go to your forearms in full plank, or drop one or both knees in forearm plank or push-up) until you are ready to commit to the quality plank or push-up. Taking regressions does not mean that you are not working hard; it simply means that you are prioritizing quality.

Listen To Your Body

Always honor your body; if you feel pain in any joint, stop the exercise immediately. Avoid exercises in which body weight is supported on the hands and in the wrists for extended periods. The plank and associated exercises in which body weight is supported by a single joint can become stressful to the wrists, elbows, and shoulder joints when performed for significant periods of time, or for a large number of repetitions. Do not perform a plank for more than four rounds in a row, which can equate to 40 to 60 seconds, as this can become stressful to joints.

Always listen to your body. If you start to feel pain or changes in your wrists or shoulders over time as you perform planks or push-ups, do not do them until you have given your body an opportunity to heal. Keep in mind that joints do not get stronger as much as the muscles around them do. So if you are working on getting stronger but you are experiencing joint pain with a particular movement, that is a sure sign that you need to back off the movement and focus on strengthening the muscles around that joint so they can support it during that movement.

Be Mindful of Changes in Blood Pressure

Certain exercises can cause drastic changes in blood pressure as a result of quick changes in body position. This is called orthostatic hypotension, and it results in compromised blood flow to the brain or working muscles. For example, moving from a plank to a jump squat too fast may cause dizziness, light-headedness, fainting, and maybe even falling, particularly when these activities are preceded by high levels of exertion. Also, when exercising early in the morning, low blood sugar levels can also cause dizziness and light-headedness. To avoid this, eat easily digested carbohydrates and simple proteins at least 2 hours before a workout. In the case of the early-morning workout, eating a combination of carbohydrates and protein that are very easy to digest (Greek yogurt) 30 minutes before working out is recommended for maximal energy and performance.

FOUNDATIONAL MOVEMENTS FOR THE CORE

Foundational movements are standardized body-weight exercises based on the ability to perform exercises as well as activities of daily living. For example, a plank is a foundational move for the core (and the upper body) that is performed in the sagittal plane. To execute the plank correctly and safely, you need to understand its purpose, which muscles should feel tension, and what a correct plank looks and feels like.

Following are descriptions of foundational core exercises that can be used in HIIT workouts, including how to execute them at the most basic level as well as additional options for added intensity. Chapter 8 describes many exercise sequence options.

Foundational Movement 1: Plank

The plank is often synonymous with core training, even eclipsing the crunch, which took the place of the sit-up in training the core. A plank is a prone (facedown) position in which the muscles are held in an isometric contraction. As described in chapter 6 on upper-body training, the plank involves maintaining a sturdy posture with the entire body weight held up on either the forearms (elbows) and toes or forefeet, or just the hands and toes or forefeet, sometimes for extended periods of time. The plank is an important isometric posture and can be very powerful in the development of core strength, proper posture, and spinal stability. As described in chapter 6, the plank can be helpful in the development of upper-body strength too. The plank keeps the spine from moving, which is exactly what core stability is designed to enhance. Using the information from chapter 6 on setting up a proper plank, let's take that information into the setup of prone (facedown) core exercises and add a few options to the basic plank.

Plank

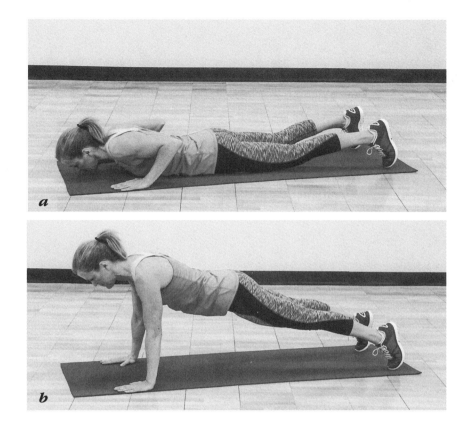

Begin by placing your hands flat on the floor with the arms close to your sides, fingers spread under the shoulder area and elbows bent and pointing directly behind the back (see figure *a*). Your legs should be straight behind you with your feet hip-width apart. Contract your abdominal muscles and tighten the quadriceps and gluteal muscles as you exhale and lift up, rising onto your toes so the balls of your feet are in contact with the floor and the heels point up (see figure *b*). Your body should be in one straight line—from the top of your head to the heels, with your body weight distributed between the hands and feet without sagging in the middle (low back or belly). Keep your eyes focused down to the floor, but hold your head up with your crown forward so the neck remains neutral.

Plank With Shoulder Tap

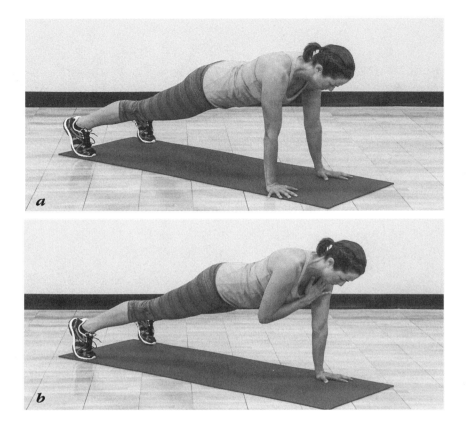

From the prone plank pose (see figure *a*), lift one hand up toward the opposite shoulder and lightly touch the shoulder joint with the fingertips (see figure *b*). Return the hand to the floor, find the plank pose once again, and repeat the tap using the other hand. Continue to alternate this opposite-hand-to-shoulder tap while maintaining core stability, trying not to allow the body to shift from side to side as you perform the tap. If you struggle with holding the hips still while performing the tap, open your feet wider for more stability.

Forearm Plank

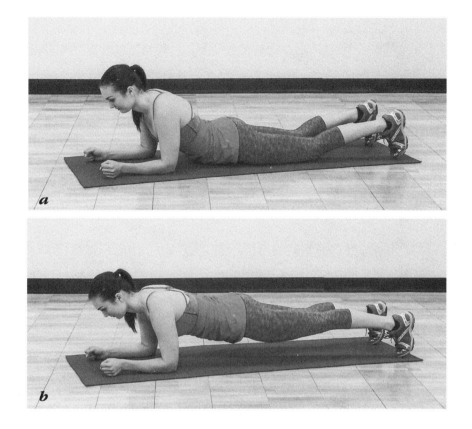

Begin by lying facedown, feet hip-width apart, and place your elbows directly under your shoulders, forearms extended with your hands in soft fists or fingers spread and hands on the floor (see figure *a*). Pull your shoulders down and away from your neck as you rise, lifting your body off the floor (see figure *b*). Your body weight should be distributed between your toes and your forearms without hiking the hips up. Keep the hands apart (as opposed to grasping them for support), and keep your elbows inside the frame of your body and parallel. Hold the abdominal wall in by bracing the anterior core muscles, and hold the body up in a long, straight line without sagging. Keep the heels pointed straight up.

Forearm Side Plank

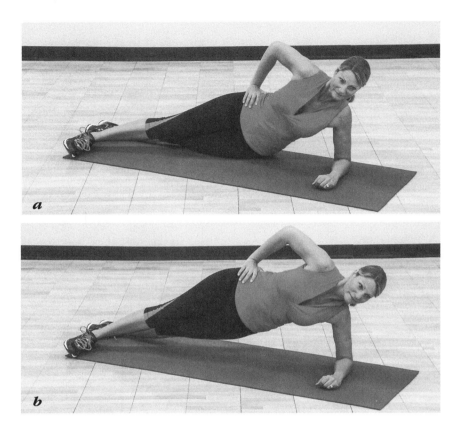

Lie on your left side with legs extended in a straight line from the hips (imagine your body as a slice of toast that has been dropped into a toaster). Place your left, flexed elbow and forearm directly under the shoulder joint with the hand extended forward from the wrist. Place the feet in a tandem stance—the top leg in front of the bottom leg, with the heel of the front foot touching and aligned with the toes of the back foot (see figure *a*). Place your right hand on top of your hip and rise up, holding up your body weight with your forearm and the sides of your feet, which are both in contact with the floor (see figure *b*). Hold the lift and then lower back down.

Plank to Pike

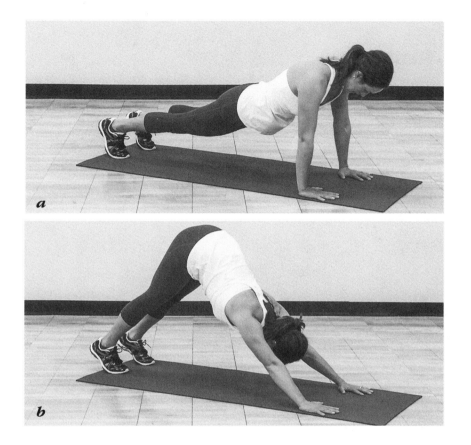

From plank pose (see figure *a*), shift your body weight up, hinging maximally at the hips and making a V-hinge position from the hips (see figure *b*). Imagine being lifted up by the hips toward the ceiling, keeping the legs straight and the spine extended. Try to keep your head between your upper arms while in the V-hinge position. Brace the abdominal wall, and then lower back into the plank with control. Continue moving back and forth from prone plank to pike. If you prefer, change the full plank to a forearm plank.

Forearm Side Plank With Reach

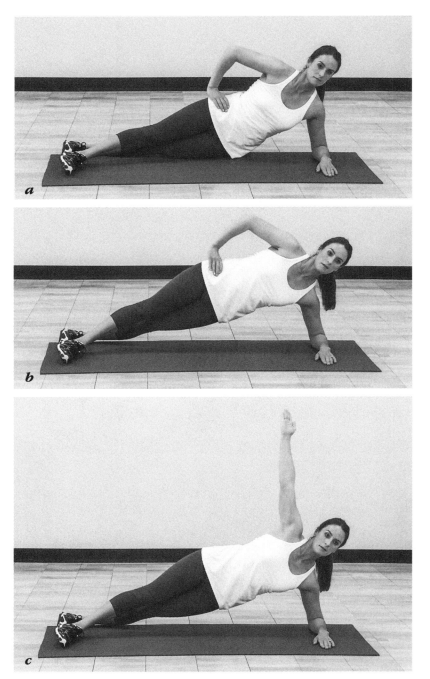

Begin on your left side with your legs extended out to the side and your left arm flexed at the elbow and directly under the shoulder joint. Place the feet in a tandem stance; the top leg is the front foot and is directly in front of the back foot (see figure *a*). Be sure the hips are stacked. Begin with your right hand on your right hip and lift your hips up into the side plank (see figure *b*); raise the hand up toward the ceiling (see figure *c*), and then lower the hand back down to the hip. Then lower the hips to the floor into the starting position. Repeat for the prescribed number of repetitions, and then switch sides.

Swimmer

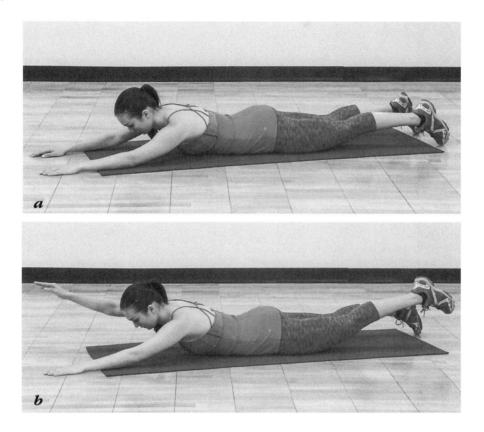

Lie facedown with your arms shoulder-width apart and extended over your head with your legs behind you, about hip-width apart (see figure *a*). Draw the abdominal wall in and stabilize the body. Lift the right arm off the floor about 3 inches (8 cm) while simultaneously lifting the left leg (thigh, knee, and foot) off the floor about 3 to 6 inches (8 to 15 cm) (see figure *b*). Continue to alternate lifting the arm and opposite leg at a controlled tempo. Keep the arms straight and the legs extended and tense as they rise and fall in controlled opposition. Lift the upper body from the shoulders and upper back and the lower body from the gluteal muscles.

Step-Back Burpee

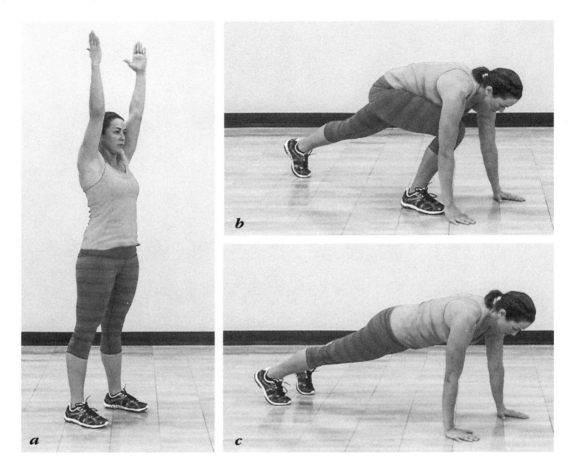

In a standing position, reach your arms overhead (see figure *a*) and then lower them to the floor just in front of your feet, stepping back one foot at a time into a plank position (see figure *b* and *c*). Hold for just a moment, and then step back in with each foot one at a time and return to an upright stance reaching your arms overhead, then repeat.

Foundational Movement 2: Supine Core Training

We are now moving into some of the supine, or faceup, core exercises including crunches, V-sits, and bridges, plus a standing exercise called a wood chop that has a similar movement pattern to a V-sit, but is performed standing. These exercises are different from the plank in terms of body position, because spinal flexion and rotation are the joint actions performed for the core. However, you will still incorporate the control and training techniques you learned for the plank with respect to maintaining a long, extended spine.

There are a few variations for the V-sit (using a medicine ball or adding rotation). Perform the moves the way that best works for your body.

V-Sit

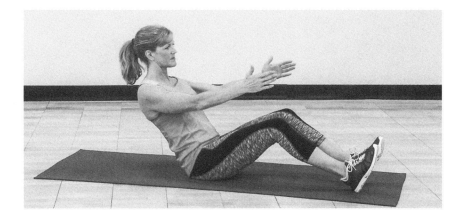

Begin by sitting on the floor with the hips flexed, knees bent, and feet about hip-width apart. Lean back, but keep your torso and spine upright. Keep the shoulders down and away from the neck. Extend the arms out, about shoulder-width apart, with the elbows extended and the fingers reaching forward. Hold the V-sit position (see figure). When you are stable, lift the feet off the floor about 3 to 6 inches (8 to 15 cm). You can make the exercise more difficult by extending the knees, straightening the legs and holding them straight to create a V shape with the torso and legs.

V-Sit With Rotation

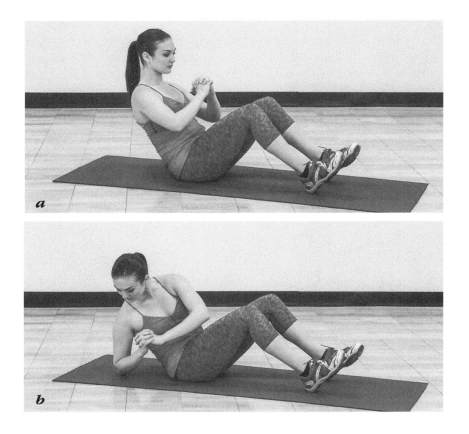

Begin by sitting on the floor with the hips flexed and the knees bent as described in the V-sit, but place the heels in light contact with the floor. Bring the hands together in a 10-finger clasp in front of the chest, elbows flexed by your sides (see figure *a*). Hold your heels in place and your spine erect as you rotate your torso, bringing the right elbow to touch the floor (see figure *b*); return to the center and rotate to the left, bringing the left elbow to the floor. Alternate the twist between the right and left sides, and maintain an upright posture using slow and controlled movements. You can make this exercise more challenging by holding a medicine ball or dumbbell.

Wood Chop

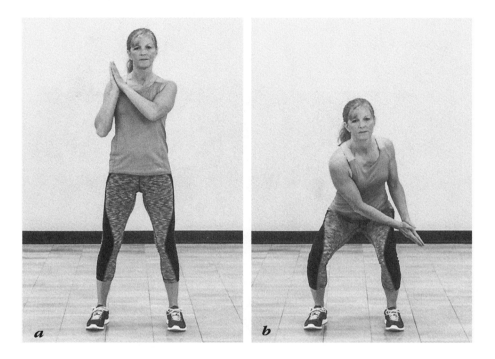

Begin in a standing position with the hands directly in front of the right shoulder, pressed together in a prayer position, creating tension between them (see figure *a*) The elbows will be apart and pointed slightly out. With feet wider than hip width and knees flexed, sit back and down into a squat posture (see figure *b*). Keeping the hands pressed together, lower them to the outside of the left knee. Be sure to stay low in the squat stance as you chop. Although you will notice a slight crunch through the torso as you perform this, try to keep the spine upright and the muscles of the torso tense and strong. Quickly bring the hands back up to the right shoulder as you stand, and continue to repeat this chopping motion, controlling the tension in the abdominal area by eliminating any unnecessary movements. Perform moves in the prescribed amount of time on the right side, and then repeat on the left. You can make this exercise more challenging by adding a squat jump or by holding a medicine ball.

▶ Eagle Wrap Reverse Crunch

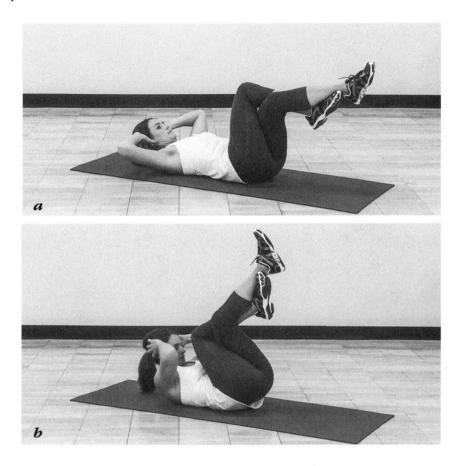

Lie on your back with your left knee pulled in toward your chest. Bring your right leg up and over the left knee, tucking the right foot under the left lower leg (see figure *a*). This is the wrap. When the legs are close together in the wrap, your top knee will align with your forehead. Bring your fingertips behind your head with the elbows pointed out. Bring the top knee toward the forehead while lifting the torso off the floor in a crunch (see figure *b*). Focus on bringing the leg closer to the forehead with every crunch. Perform a set with the right leg over the left and then another set with the left leg over the right.

Half Bicycle Crunch

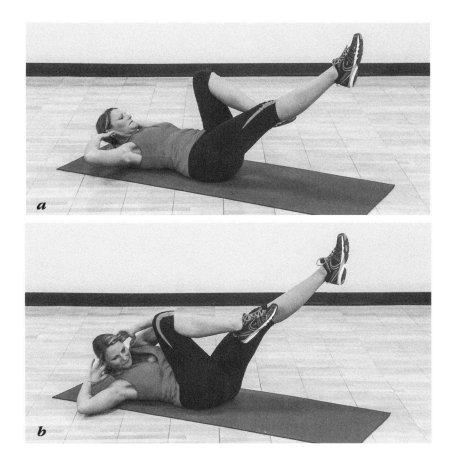

Begin on your back, drawing your left knee into your chest and extending your right leg so that the left foot is aligned with the right knee of the extended leg (see figure *a*). Place your fingertips lightly behind your ears on the base of your skull, elbows pointing out. Twist through your center, bringing the left elbow to touch the right knee (see figure *b*). Lower your shoulders and head to the floor, and extend the right leg while simultaneously pulling the left knee into the chest. Continue to alternate—pull the right knee up and touch with the left elbow, and then pull the left knee up while lowering the upper body to the floor. The leg pattern is called a switch. Touch only the right knee to the left elbow for the half bicycle crunch right, but perform the leg switch each time. Repeat using the left knee touching the right elbow for the half bicycle crunch left.

▶ Full Bicycle Crunch

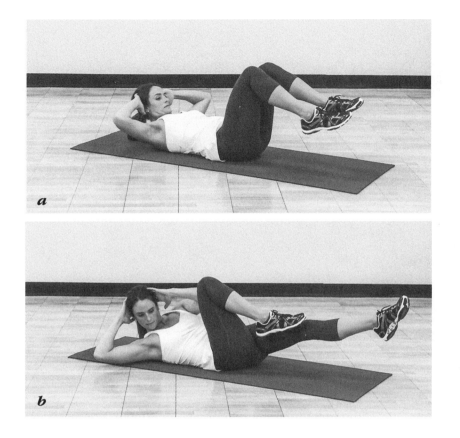

Begin on your back, drawing your knees into your chest (see figure *a*). Place your fingertips lightly behind your ears on the base of your skull, elbows pointing out. Twist through your center, bringing the left elbow to touch the right knee, as you extend the left leg and then extend the right leg while simultaneously pulling the left knee into the chest and touching the right elbow to the left knee (see figure *b*). The leg pattern is called the switch; it is the same as that described in the half bicycle crunch. Continue to alternate—pull the right knee up and touch it with the left elbow, and then pull the left knee up and touch it with the right elbow. Continue to alternate, bringing the right elbow to the left knee and the left elbow to the right knee. Be precise with the foot-to-knee contact to create more tension in the anterior core and abdominal area.

Bridge

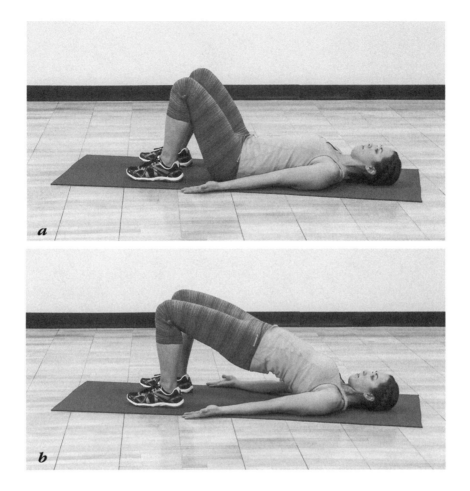

Lie on your back with your feet hip-width apart and your head and shoulders relaxed. Extend your arms out on the floor, reaching toward the heels with palms faceup (see figure *a*). This will guide you in foot placement relative to your body length. Lift your hips as high as possible, squeezing your gluteals as you drive the hips up. Keep your shoulders and neck relaxed and your chin tucked (see figure *b*). Pause at the top, and then lower to the floor and repeat.

▶ Single-Leg Bridge

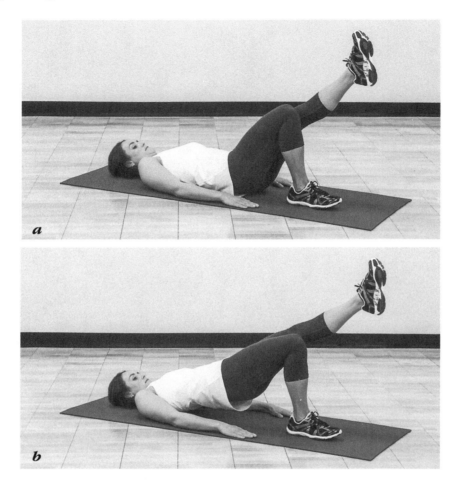

Lie on your back with your feet hip-width apart and your head and shoulders relaxed. Extend your arms out on the floor, reaching toward the heels. This will guide you in foot placement relative to your body length. Center your right foot, and lift and extend your left leg, holding it up and off the floor but attempting to place your knees parallel to each other (see figure *a*). Maintain tension in the thigh of the extended leg as you lift the hips up and off the floor as high as possible (see figure *b*). Squeeze the gluteals and drive the hips up, and then lower the hips, but maintain the lift in the extended leg and repeat the hip lift. Once the recommended time is up, switch legs.

Chapter 8 combines the lower-body, upper-body, and core exercises into workout segments from which you can choose to create the perfect exercise combination for every workout. The exercises are organized into a menu of options and further broken down into max intervals, mixed intervals, and hard, harder, hardest categories. This will allow you to easily choose exercises based on body-part focus, equipment availability, work intensity, and the time frame you have in which to work out. Chapter 8 also covers appropriate exercise progressions and regressions, or techniques and strategies you can use to make the exercises more or less intense based on your particular needs.

We also examine in chapter 8 which exercises create the immediate HIIT factor, why some exercises work better together than others, and how to use strategy and planning to get through each workout using the highest quality of movement. Only by making the highest commitment to your workouts will you achieve the results you are looking for.

SELECTING YOUR EXERCISES

Now that we have considered the many exercises that can be used for HIIT workouts, let's take a look at how to put them together to create tailored workouts to meet your HIIT program goals. We begin with a discussion of creating high intensity right from the start. The exercise sequences that follow are organized into max interval and mixed interval Tabata sequences and hard, harder, hardest interval sequences. Each exercise menu is organized by time frames with a precise training emphasis and includes exercises for the upper body, lower body, and core, plus equipment options. The exercise options and movement patterns are grouped so you can easily select exercises that complement one another and provide intensity, effectiveness, and above all, safety. Although these exercises build intensity rather quickly, our focus is always on performance, not simply fatigue.

Always remember that the quality of your movements is far more important than the quantity. This chapter also explains how to make every movement matter, emphasizing that any fitness level can be successful using these training techniques.

CREATING AN IMMEDIATE HIIT

Because HIIT workouts involve short-duration, high-intensity microbursts of activity followed by shorter bouts of active or passive recovery, it is crucial that you choose movements that offer an immediate feeling of intensity and effort. The exercises need to create fatigue that is cumulative over the short duration. Even though the workouts may be only 2 to 4 minutes long, they should be the hardest 2 to 4 minutes of training you can possibly do! Therefore, as the volume of training increases, your efforts should also increase. For this to occur, you need a good understanding of which exercises create an immediate high-intensity effort and which exercise qualities to look for.

Although there are hundreds of choices in addition to those presented here, this chapter simplifies the selection process by describing the qualities a HIIT exercise should contain. Let's take a moment to review two interval formats from chapter 3 (Tabata and hard, harder, hardest).

As described in chapter 3, a max interval is a four-minute Tabata interval using one exercise for maximal intensity and effort. A hard, harder, hardest interval consists of three rounds of the following timing: 40 Seconds of work followed by 20 seconds of rest; 30 seconds of work with 15 seconds of rest; and 20 seconds of work with only 10 seconds of rest. So the mixed and max intervals consist of 8 rounds, and the hard, harder, hardest intervals consist of 3 rounds. The training intensity is so high that you will not be able to complete more than one max interval in a single workout. If you can, consider increasing the exercise intensity by using the progression options in chapter 9.

As you recall, max interval training involves performing *one exercise* for 20 seconds at extreme intensity (i.e., about 170 percent of V\od\O$_2$max) followed by 10 seconds of rest. This is repeated for 4 minutes, totaling eight rounds, or cycles. The max interval represents maximal intensity, or the hardest Tabata protocol you can perform. This approach takes your body to failure as you cross the anaerobic threshold and become extremely fatigued and breathless. In HIIT programs, max intervals are used primarily for muscular power and anaerobic cardio. To qualify as a max interval, exercise should meet the following criteria:

Simple Movements

The joint actions that drive these powerful max-interval movements must be simple to follow, keeping in mind that sometimes less is more. Less complexity in patterns and movements creates less confusion, and simple, powerful exercises are easier to progress and regress, or make more or less manageable, as fatigue overwhelms you.

Major Muscle and Compound Movements

The movement patterns should demonstrate triple flexion. This refers to joint actions or movement at the ankles, knees, and hips. Typically, when these joints are acting simultaneously, the movement is simple and powerful and the largest muscles of the body are likely engaged. When the ankles, knees, and hips are working together, they create vigorous, compound movements requiring significant amounts of energy, which will likely make you breathless.

Bigger and Slower May be Better

Larger ranges of motion performed more slowly may offer you a bigger bang for your buck. Sometimes more energy is needed to move with decreased speed and control, so consider the speed and size of your movements when you are working toward fatigue.

As a general rule, strength movements performed slowly are more challenging, and cardio-based movements performed quickly are more challenging. For example, squat jumps with an elbow drive performed with perfect form and technique can build more strength if executed more slowly and with plenty of control. Use speed for more anaerobic intensity as long as you are still able to control the movement.

Immediate HIIT Factor

The exercises selected for max intervals must create a fatigue response right away. This is not to say that the first or second repetition, or even the first or second round, of the movement should cause you to bend over in breathlessness, but by round 2 or 3, you should notice that the exercise is a challenge, and you should be bordering on crossing, if not almost at or about to cross, your anaerobic threshold. If this is not the case, you are either not working hard enough, or the exercise is not appropriate for a max interval.

Goal Oriented and Standardized

Each of the exercises presented in this book involves a specific action to which you are accountable. For example, for the squat jump with elbow drive, every squat requires that the tips of the elbows make contact with the legs, touching just above the knees when down in the squat. When jumping up, the elbows should drive back and behind the body. These features help to standardize the move, creating accountability for each squat and jump performed. If the squat is done without touching the tips of the elbows to the tops of the knee area, or the elbows fail to drive back and behind the body on the jump, the movement should be slowed down until each repetition meets the criteria. This ensures that your movements are standardized to ensure quality over quantity. It also ensures that you are performing each movement to the best of your ability.

Progressive and Regressive Options

People at all fitness levels should be able to experience every move without limitation for the full duration of the interval. This is why it is important that you choose moves that you can easily regress (make easier or more manageable) or progress (make more challenging and difficult) without significant transition. Therefore, any exercise that is vigorous and can ramp up in intensity very quickly will work for this training program. Chapter 9 offers much more on this subject.

For example, burpees, cycle lunges, speedskaters, and jumping jacks can all be tough, but they can also be regressed so you can finish all eight rounds without putting yourself at risk of injury or quitting. We focus on this very important aspect of HIIT exercise selection in chapter 9.

EXERCISE SELECTION MENUS

We begin with a menu for max intervals (figure 8.1), then offer a menu of mixed intervals (figure 8.2), and end with a hard, harder, hardest menu (figure 8.3). Although the mixed interval and hard, harder, hardest protocols are not as intense as the max interval protocol, they are important for overall training and to provide movement variety to create a complete HIIT workout experience.

Chapters 5, 6, and 7 provide descriptions of the exercises for the lower-body, upper-body, and core, respectively. In the following menus, we combine the exercises in such a way that you can choose the movements you want to use for your workouts. The workout combinations in chapter 10 are just examples—you can pick out your own exercises from these menus and replace those used in the workouts in chapter 10. They're designed so that you can interchange exercises for endless workout possibilities.

Keep in mind that you can select two max interval workouts from the menu and create your own mixed interval, and you will see mixed interval options that are simply a combination of two max intervals. Even though you are offered specific combinations here, you can mix and match as you choose.

Figure 8.1 Max Interval Menu

1	2	3	4	5	6
Squat with elbow drive: p.48	Quarter-turn squat: p.51	Two-knee push-up: p.91	Side-to-side squat: p.52	Plié squat: p.53	Squat jack: p.55
7	8	9	10	11	12
Wood chop squat: p.56	Burpee: p.57	Front to back lunge: p.59	Cycle lunge: p.60	Diagonal lunge with floor touch: p.61	Brazilian lunge: p.62
13	14	15	16	17	18
Messy lunge: p.63	Curtsy lunge: p.65	Lateral lunge with adduction: p.67	Front lunge with knee lift: p.68	Pendulum lunge: p.69	Dolphin push-up: p.73
19	20	21	22	23	24
Mountain climber: p.72	Single-leg squat: p.50	Mogul twist: p.75	Twist: p.76	Power speed skip: p.77	Jumping jack with arms to front: p.78
25	26	27	28	29	30
Basic lunge: p.58	Plié squat with heel click: p.54	Squat jump: p.47	Burpee with vertical jump: p.70	Speedskater: p.74	Plank to pike: p.123

Figure 8.2 Mixed Interval Menu

1	2	3	4	5	6
Basic squat: p.45 basic lunge: p.58	Plank: p.87 one-knee push-up: p.92	Forearm plank: p.121 forearm side plank: p.122	Single-leg squat: p.50 cycle lunge: p.60	Bent-over row: p.98 biceps curl: p.107	V-sit: p.127 full bicycle crunch: p.132
7	8	9	10	11	12
Squat jack: p.55 Brazilian lunge: p.62	Shoulder press: p.101 military-style push-up: p.90	Wood chop squat: p.56 mountain climber: p.72	Side-to-side squat: p.52 squat to heel raise: p.46	Chest press: p.93 lat pulldown: p.96	Half bicycle crunch (left and right): p.131 full bicycle crunch: p.132
13	14	15	16	17	18
Offset stance squat: p.49 lateral lunge with touch: p.66	Seated row: p.100 single-arm biceps curl: p.108	Bridge: p.133 single-leg bridge: p.134	Quarter-turn squat: p.51 messy lunge: p.63	Push press: p.102 quadruped triceps press: p.110	Plank: p.87 dolphin push-up: p.73
19	20	21	22	23	24
Plié squat: p.53 single-leg balance lunge: p.64	Forearm side plank with reach: p.124 triceps push-up: p.89	Swimmer: p.125 plank with shoulder tap: p.120	Curtsy lunge: p.65 twist: p.76	Basic push-up: p.88 step-back burpee: p.126	Bridge: p.133 full bicycle crunch: p.132
25	26	27	28	29	30
Speedskater: p.74 squat jump: p.47	Single-arm bent-over row: p.99 upright row with dumbbells: p.103	V-sit with rotation: p.128 eagle wrap reverse crunch: p.130	Jumping jack with arms to front: p.78 mogul twist: p.75	Chest fly: p.95 single-arm pulldown: p.97	Wood chop: p.129 plank to pike: p.123

Figure 8.3 Hard, Harder, Hardest Menu

1	2	3	4	5	6
Basic squat: p.45 squat to heel raise: p.46 squat jump: p.47	Plank: p.87 plank with shoulder tap: p.120 one-knee push-up: p.92	V-sit: p.127 V-sit with rotation: p.128 full bicycle crunch: p.132	Lateral lunge with touch: p.66 lateral lunge with adduction: p.67 pendulum lunge: p.69	Basic push-up: p.88 chest press: p.93 triceps kickback: p.109	Wood chop: p.129 step-back burpee: p.126 Jumping jack with arms to front: p.78
7	8	9	10	11	12
Brazilian lunge: p.62 messy lunge: p.63 front to back lunge: p.59	Chest press: p.93 two-knee push-up: p.91 chest fly: p.95	Swimmer: p.125 bridge: p.133 single-leg bridge: p.134	Squat jack: p.55 burpee: p.57 plank with shoulder tap: p.120	Lat pulldown: p.96 single-arm pulldown: p.97 upright row with tubing: p.104	Plank to pike: p.123 half bicycle crunch (left and right): p.131
13	14	15	16	17	18
Squat to heel raise: p.46 squat with elbow drive: p.48 plié squat: p.54	Military-style push-up: p.90 seated row: p.100 lateral raise with tubing: p.106	Power speed skip: p.77 wood chop: p.129 V-sit: p.127	Diagonal lunge with floor touch: p.61 curtsy lunge: p.65 twist: p.76	Biceps curl: p.107 single-arm biceps curl: p.108 lateral raise with dumbbells: p.105	Half bicycle crunch (left and right): p.131 full bicycle crunch: p.132
19	20	21	22	23	24
Jumping jack with arms to front: p.78 mogul twist: p.75 speedskater: p.74	Shoulder press: p.101 biceps curl: p.107 single-arm biceps curl: p.108	Full bicycle crunch: p.132 bridge: p.133 eagle wrap reverse crunch: p.130	Cycle lunge: p.60 basic squat: p.45 plié squat with heel click: p.54	Chest press: p.93 triceps push-up: p.89 plank: p.87	Dolphin push-up: p.73 forearm side plank: p.122 plank to pike: p.123
25	26	27	28	29	30
Burpee with vertical jump: p.70 basic lunge: p.58 single-leg balance lunge: p.64	Single-arm bent-over row: p.99 upright row with dumbbells: p.103 single-arm biceps curl: p.108	Mountain climber: p.72 plank: p.87 forearm side plank with reach: p.124	Front lunge with knee lift: p.68 messy lunge: p.63 twist: p.76	Burpee with push-up: p.71 chest press: p.93 lat pulldown: p.96	Wood chop squat: p.56 V-sit with rotation: p.128 single-leg bridge: p.134

*For sequences with a right and a left lead, perform twice or alternate to balance the muscle groups and body parts.

Now that you are acquainted with the exercises described in chapters 5, 6, and 7, and the menu of exercises here, chapter 9 will help you choose progressive and regressive options for maximal success, select equipment options to apply to the exercises, and decide how to monitor your timing. Chapter 10 offers workouts in 20-, 30-, and 45-minute sequences that focus on specific body parts and equipment to add variety and to meet specific training goals.

HIGH-INTENSITY INTERVAL WORKOUTS

PLANNING YOUR WORKOUT

This chapter provides recommendations for mixing and matching exercises and using regressions, progressions, and modifications in the exercises you choose. You will learn how to time your workouts and how to use equipment with the exercises presented in chapters 5, 6, and 7.

All exercises can be scaled up or down in intensity so you can successfully complete each exercise sequence. Strategies and techniques described in this chapter can be applied at any time to create continuous, flowing sequences. You will need to plan your exercise regressions to best meet your training needs without compromising your safety. The goal is to be able to maintain control through the hard parts so you do not have to stop when the workloads become intense. The training in this book is designed to make you ultrafit by progressively applying the principle of overload.

We also look at timing options so you can stay on task with minimal disruption or confusion. You will learn how to prepare for your workouts, including getting the equipment you need and using specific tools and toys.

SCALING THE MOVEMENT PATTERNS

HIIT requires that you work as hard as you can as soon as you begin, not wait for round 3 or 4 to turn it on. For example, after you warm up, you perform an exercise sequence to failure. This means that you try as hard as you can to get as fatigued as possible at the beginning of the exercise sequence. You then have a rest period (maybe 10 seconds, maybe longer), after which you repeat this maximal effort. You need to choose movements that don't build in intensity, but rather, those that feel very intense right away. Your strategies for progressions and regressions will help you get through all the intervals, especially when you feel as though you can't.

The following techniques will help you manage your accumulating fatigue. Stopping or quitting (unless there is pain or potential for injury) is not an encouraged option. Using these approaches to manage the overload is the key to sustaining the movements, even in the face of overwhelming fatigue.

On-Ramps and Off-Ramps

Because all exercises must be achievable, you need built-in on-ramps (ways to make exercises more challenging) and off-ramps (ways to make exercises less intense) so that you can complete each round without stopping. Consider the speedskater exercise. You could decrease the intensity by slowing down, making the range of motion smaller, or shortening the distance between you and the floor by placing a cone or other object in front of you to touch. This way you maintain uniformity and quality in the execution of the exercise. This guideline refers to the quality of movement over the quantity. Performing more repetitions does not necessarily equate to better fitness outcomes. High-quality movements produce high-quality training results.

Speed

If the movements become too overwhelming or unsustainable, simply slow down. This can be done without stopping.

Range of Motion

Changing the size of the movement pattern can often make the exercise more manageable. Generally, smaller ranges of motion decrease intensity, but this is not always the case. For example, a mogul twist can be made very challenging by slowing down and sitting into the movement. It can also be made more challenging by going faster, which creates a different type of fatigue.

Base of Support

Stability is a function of the body's natural base of support and its own center of gravity. For example, when standing, for most people, the center of gravity is right around the middle of the body, and the base of support is related to foot placement. Maximal stability occurs when the center of gravity is within the base of support. When the base of support is decreased, the center of gravity may move beyond the base, making movement more challenging. For example, bringing the feet close together or standing on one leg challenges stability much more than standing with the feet set wide apart. Additionally, holding a plank pose or performing a push-up with the feet side by side is more difficult than having a wide foot position or one knee down. And having hand position that is wider than shoulder width for a plank or push-up would be more manageable than having a narrow hand position. A strategy for decreasing intensity, or creating an off-ramp, would be to stand wider, widen the hand positions, or drop a knee during a plank or push-up.

Holding Postures

Sometimes, during a movement, your body will fatigue and you may believe you cannot do another repetition, but you can. You can hold your body in one part of the exercise and actively rest while mentally encouraging yourself to keep going. For example, the push-up has an up and a down phase. At the top of the range is the plank phase, and at the bottom is a very high-intensity position in which the triceps, chest, and core have to stabilize the body when the muscles are contracted and under tremendous tension to keep the body from dropping to the floor. When you are feeling fatigued during push-ups, you can hold the top of the push-up position, or the plank, and not perform another push-up until you are ready. You can even drop a knee to create a larger base of support while you hold the position. This is not the same as stopping because your muscles are still actively engaged in the movement. It may be true that you can't perform another push-up until you have time to rest, but using this holding technique, you are still working the muscles without compromising your workout or your safety.

Increasing or Decreasing Impact

Jumping and other activities that involve leaving the floor can be very challenging for some people. Adding impact to a movement definitely increases the intensity because the body must work against gravity. However, impact is not right for everybody; joint issues and other preexisting conditions may prohibit some people from adding a jump to a particular exercise. Also, as fatigue sets in, sustaining a jump may not be feasible. It is perfectly fine to take the jump out of a movement pattern, either completely if it is not a safe way to increase intensity, or just for a few repetitions if the workloads are becoming too intense. A progressive method is to perform a couple of jumps in a row and then go back to the nonimpact method, and then add jumps when you feel as though you can withstand the impact. This can be done in a single interval (20 seconds) or even within an entire 4-minute sequence (e.g., add the jumping movements for rounds 1 and 2, but take them out for round 3, and then see if you can add them back in for round 4).

GUIDELINES FOR SETTING UP YOUR EXERCISES

Max intervals typically rely strictly on body weight where mixed intervals use a combination of body weight and portable equipment. When using either max or mixed intervals, keep the following guidelines in mind to maintain high levels of intensity and timing consistency, so your workouts flow seamlessly.

Preparing for Workouts

Because of the short duration of both the exercises and the recovery periods, you have very little time between them. Therefore, it is very important to prepare for each sequence before the workout begins. Have all the equipment you need available to grab in the short time between sequences.

Exercise Order

When using max intervals, exercise order is irrelevant because you are performing only one exercise. However, with mixed intervals and the hard, harder, hardest protocol, you need to follow a few guidelines to ensure that you know exactly which exercise to perform when.

- *Mixed intervals*: Perform exercise 1 for rounds 1 and 2; perform exercise 2 for rounds 3 and 4; perform exercise 1 again for rounds 5 and 6; and then perform exercise 2 again for rounds 7 and 8.
- *Hard, harder, hardest*: Start with the larger muscles, and finish with the smaller muscles. For example, for a chest sequence, begin with a push-up for 40 seconds and then perform a forearm side plank for 30 seconds. Finish with a triceps exercise for 20 seconds. This way, the larger, stabilizing muscles will not be prematurely fatigued, and you will be able to safely perform the entire sequence with precision.

Lead Leg Changes

In a mixed interval, in which you perform exercise 1 for rounds 1 and 2, if there is a right leg and a left leg change, start with and stay on one lead leg. The next time you switch back to the first exercise, change lead legs. For example, in a mixed interval consisting of a Brazilian lunge and a twist, rounds 1 and 2 would consist of Brazilian lunges leading with the right leg. Rounds 3 and 4 would consist of exercise 2, the twist. In rounds 5 and 6, you would perform the Brazilian lunge again, but this time leading with the left leg. You would then complete the mixed interval by performing the twist for rounds 7 and 8. This maintains high levels of intensity while decreasing confusion to help you stay on track with your goal of completing all rounds using both legs.

Staying on Task

It is really important that you work through your entire interval. For example, if the work bout is 20 seconds long, you need to keep going until the entire 20-second period is over. If rest is for 10 seconds, then you only have 10 seconds to rest and prepare for your next round.

Recovery Between Intervals

Recovery time between the interval sequences will vary, but it is recommended that you follow the 2:1 ratio. For example, if you are performing a 4-minute Tabata sequence, then a 2-minute recovery between intervals is recommended.

TIMING YOUR SEQUENCES

Using a timer to define your rest and work intervals for HIIT workouts or any timed circuit is ideal. Options include many downloadable applications for smartphones and other electronic devices, a stopwatch or clock, or preprogrammed music.

Downloadable Applications

Many Tabata timers are available free and for purchase as downloadable applications from the Internet. These timers are very easy to use and can be interfaced with your smartphone, iPad, or computer. Choose a timer that offers you lead time and clear, distinct indicators (bells, whistles, or other sounds) to indicate the start and end of a round and a full 4-minute Tabata sequence. Many applications offer the option to change the timing sequences, the sounds, and the colors that indicate changes. Two options can be found at www.intervaltimer.com and at www.beach-fitness.com/tabata-timer.

Stopwatch or Clock

A stopwatch or clock with a second hand can help you time your HIIT workouts. Be sure to have the timepiece in your immediate view so you can stay on task.

Prerecorded Music

Research has consistently demonstrated that music has a profound effect on athletes' ability to work though discomfort. In fact, music can actually help with movement rhythm and pace and can even distract you from the perceived exertion. Several fitness music companies offer both downloads and CDs for use with HIIT protocols. These

CDs or playlists are easy to play through a stereo or computer or can be downloaded to a smartphone or iPad. The music can help maintain intensity and motivation.

Dynamix Music (www.dynamixmusic.com) offers six music playlists for use in HIIT workouts. Tabata Bootcamp Volumes 1, 3, and 5 offer sequences in 20/10 Tabata timing. Volumes 2, 4, and 6 (www.tabatabootcamp.com) offer timing in the hard, harder, hardest timing sequences (40, 30, and 20 seconds). Power Music (www.powermusic.com) and Yes! Fitness Music (www.yesfitnessmusic.com) also offer interval timing sequences that will help you control your training sessions with audible cues so you will not have to watch a clock or stopwatch.

EQUIPMENT OPTIONS AND SELECTION

Using tools and portable equipment for HIIT workouts is a great way to change up your routines, increase the intensity of training, target specific areas of the body, and promote longevity in your workouts. Chapters 5, 6, and 7 present a variety of lower-body, upper-body, and core exercises that can easily incorporate equipment. Following are ideas for using equipment with specific exercises:

- Hold dumbbells, a medicine ball, or a kettlebell, or use a suspension trainer, for almost any squat or lunge for the lower body and in many of the upper-body exercises.
- Tubing can be incorporated into the following upper-body exercises: standing chest press, shoulder press, biceps curl, triceps press, and lat pulldown.
- The medicine ball can be helpful when performing any rotational movement for the core or integrated into many of the lower-body exercises.
- The mini-trampoline is extremely helpful in the Tabata protocols, because you can create significant intensity without having to sustain ground reaction forces and impact.
- Gliding disks are easily used under the hands and knees, in plank pose, and under the feet in lunges, burpees, and bridges.

Now that you have a thorough understanding of the exercises, how to time your workouts, and strategies for overcoming fatigue, let's take a look at the workouts in chapter 10.

HIIT WORKOUTS

Now that you have an understanding of the HIIT concept, the way the body responds to this type of training, and the kinds of exercises that are ideal, let's take a look at the best HIIT routines to fit into any busy schedule.

This chapter presents five 20-minute workouts, six 30-minute workouts, and five 45-minute workouts. You will also find an easy-to-use template for creating your own HIIT workouts using the exercise menus provided in chapter 8. Suggestions for warm-up and cool-down routines are also included, as well as 30 max-interval 4-minute microburst workouts you can do any day of the week to incinerate calories and keep yourself on track with your weight loss goals and fitness routine.

Each workout includes body weight and equipment options and a time frame so you will know exactly how long it will take you to perform it. The create-your-own workout template will help you customize your workouts. Finally, several max interval Tabata sequences provide very quick and effective options for fitting one 4-minute Tabata routine into your day regardless of how much time you have to exercise or how fit you are. Even though consecutive HIIT workouts are not recommended daily, these 4-minute sequences are short enough to simply add a boost to your daily caloric expenditure. The 4-minute Tabata sequences are also ideal for increasing your level of fitness. If you are not yet ready to implement an entire HIIT workout, the 4-minute sequences performed daily and integrated into your current routine will help you build up to a full HIIT workout.

ACTIVE RECOVERY WORKOUTS

HIIT protocols are not recommended for daily exercise because the intensity is so high that you need time to recover. This is why recovery workouts are so important when using HIIT protocols. Active recovery by this definition does not mean no exercise; it means exercising, but doing something other than a super-hard HIIT workout.

Active recovery workouts can take a variety of forms, as long as you are not crossing your anaerobic threshold. Following are some suggestions. You can perform these workouts on the days between your HIT workouts. Keep the intensity comfortable, and perform them for anywhere from 20 minutes to an hour.

- Treadmill walking or jogging
- Elliptical trainer
- Recumbent cycling or cycling class
- Zumba, step, or other low-impact aerobic fitness activity or class
- Swimming or aquatic fitness class
- Yoga
- Pilates

WARMING UP AND COOLING DOWN

Preparing your body for your workout with a proper warm-up is vital to ensure effectiveness and safety. No matter what type of exercise you perform, a warm-up should never be neglected.

Warm Up Before You Work Out

No matter which workout you choose, it is always necessary to warm up beforehand. The warm-up should take anywhere from 3 to 10 minutes, depending on the workout and how you are feeling. As a result of your warm-up, your body will respond to the exercises better through increased body temperature, blood flow, and hormone release, all of which prepare the body for exercise. Also, your risk of injury is significantly reduced when you warm up before you exercise.

Your warm-up options include a light-intensity cardio activity such as walking in place, treadmill walking, or jogging; using an elliptical trainer or recumbent cycle; or anything that lubricates the joints, increases body temperature and blood flow, and causes you to feel warmer and more agile. You can also perform body-weight exercises such as squats or lunges with decreased range of motion to rehearse the movements you will be performing in your workout. Rhythmic flexibility movements may also be very effective in getting the body ready for a great workout.

Try the following preworkout warm-up that focuses on body weight and range of motion and includes fast-paced but flowing movements for improved agility and mobility.

PRE-HIIT WORKOUT WARM-UP

Seated Ankle Plantarflexion and Dorsiflexion

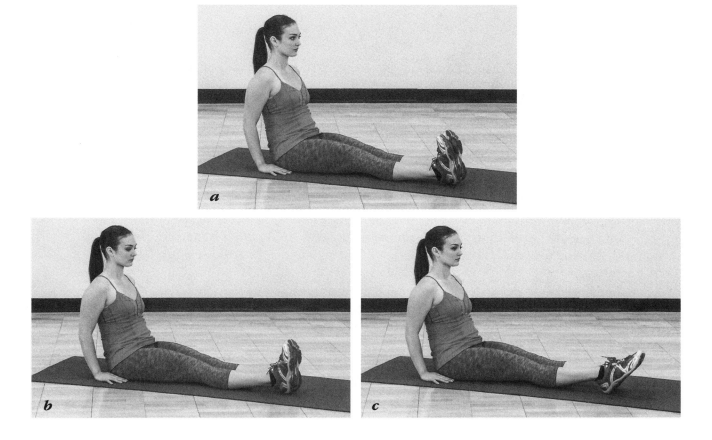

Sit tall with your legs extended in front of you. Point and flex your ankles (see figures
a-c). You can also rotate your ankles in a circle 10 times.

Active Leg Raise

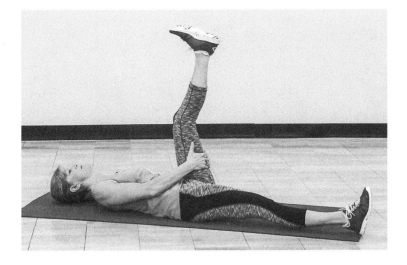

Lie on your back and alternate bringing the knees into the chest. Straighten the legs and use one hand to lift one leg up (straight knee). Bring the leg closer to the body by placing the hands behind the thigh and gently pulling the leg (see figure). Perform this move five times, and then do the same on the other leg, not holding the stretch more than two to five seconds each.

Seated Shoulder Reach

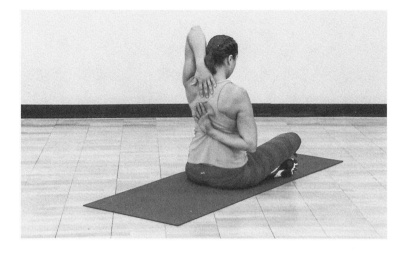

From a seated position, reach your hands behind your back. Alternating one hand up and the other down, attempt to touch your hands behind your back (see figure). Alternate arms five times each.

Seated Figure-Four Position

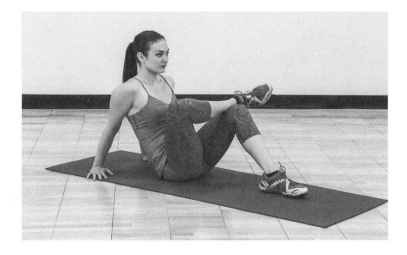

Alternate bringing the right knee over the left thigh, with the bottom knee flexed (see figure), and then switch. Maintain a continuous rhythm, pressing the hands into the floor each time you switch legs.

Cobra to Child's Pose

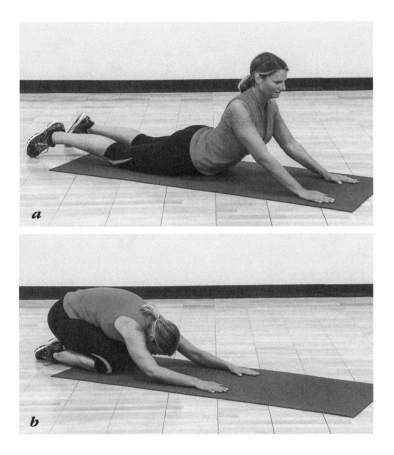

Lie facedown, relaxing the entire body on the floor, and use the arms to press the upper body up and off the floor by pressing onto the hands, arching the back, and lifting the chest (see figure *a*). Fully extend the arms if possible, or press as high as you can and then relax back into a child's pose, bringing the hips to the heels with the arms extended in front of you (see figure *b*). Perform this sequence five times.

Quadruped Shoulder Reach With Creep

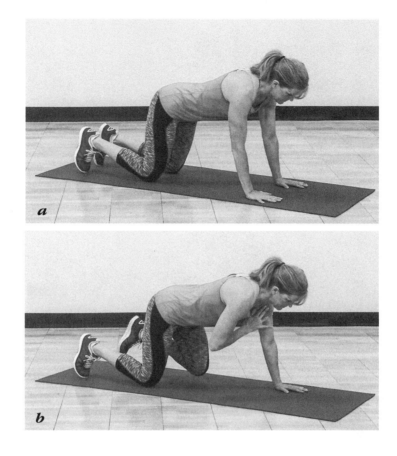

From a hands-and-knees position (see figure *a*), reach up with your right hand to touch your left shoulder while simultaneously lifting the left knee a few inches (around 7 cm) from the floor and slowly creeping forward (see figure *b*). Perform five times on each side, alternating.

Squat to Push-Up

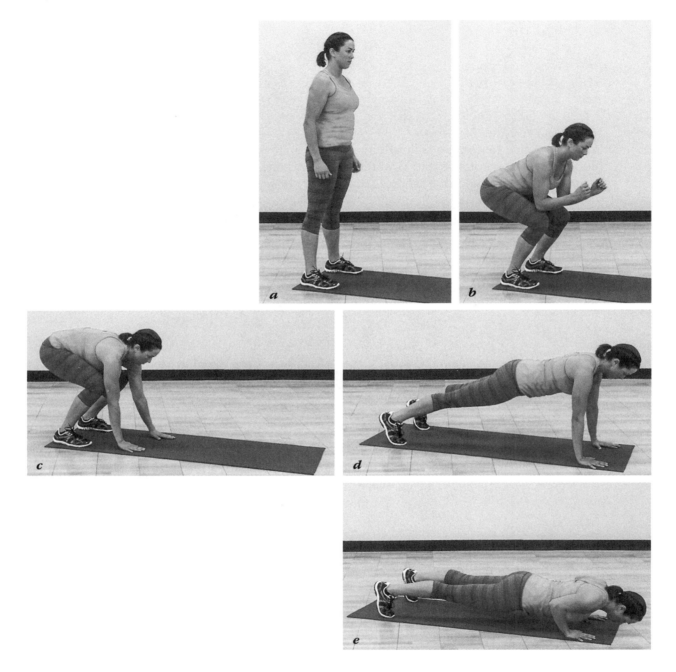

From a standing position (see figure *a*), lower into a deep squat (see figure *b*) and then place your hands on the floor and walk your hands forward until you are in a plank pose (see figure *c* and *d*). Perform one push-up (see figure *e*), and then use your hands to walk back to your feet, rising up first into a deep squat and then back to standing. Do five times total.

Cool Down and Transition Out

To transition out of the exercise session, you will want to bring your body back to as close to a preexercise, or resting, state as possible. Once you are finished with your last HIIT interval, begin by slowing down, but not stopping movement completely. This is important because slowing down gradually allows the muscles to continue to pump blood through the body, thus decreasing the chances of significant changes in blood pressure, which could cause light-headedness or even fainting. This can be done with a march in place or a side-to-side touch. Also, a gradual reduction in speed and movement intensity lowers the heart rate to resting levels and puts the body on notice that you are finished requiring increased oxygen uptake, increased blood flow, water for sweat to cool the body, and energy production.

Stretching at the end of a workout is also very beneficial because the muscles are warm and pliable and therefore more prepared for static (held) stretches. In fact, it is recommended that you perform static stretching postworkout rather than preworkout.

Take 3 to 5 minutes to bring your body back down to resting levels. A sure sign that you have not allowed enough time to cool down and transition out of the workout is continued sweating. If you are finished with your workout, but are still sweating, your postworkout routine was too short; you need to spend a little more time transitioning out of the workout before moving on with your day.

Try the following cool-down, or transition, sequence postworkout. Use control and stay in each stretch for at least 10 seconds, focusing on your breath, muscles, and joint ranges of motion.

POST-HIIT WORKOUT COOL-DOWN

Back-Lying Knee to Chest

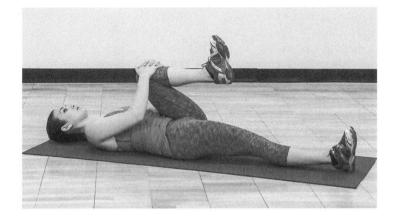

Lie on your back, lengthening your right leg and pulling the left knee up into your chest (see figure). Use your hands to create a 10-finger grip, and inhale and exhale as you continue to pull the knee closer to your body. Exhale and pull in three times. Repeat on the other side.

Straight-Leg Raise

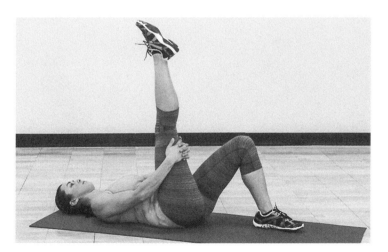

While lying on your back, flex the left knee and place the left foot on the floor while using your hands to pull your straight right leg upward (see figure). Point the right toe and inhale and exhale as you gently attempt to pull the leg a little closer. Hold each stretch for about 10 seconds. Repeat on the other side.

Supine Figure Four

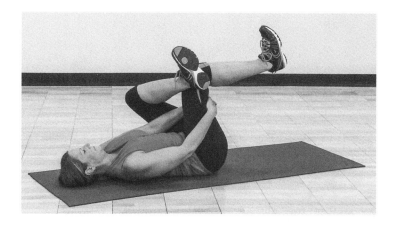

In a back-lying position, bend one knee and cross the other over it. Reach your hands through your bent knee and thigh and grasp the back of the hamstring or the top of the knee joint and pull the leg closer to the body (see figure). You can use your elbow to create more leverage. Hold the stretch, feeling the intensity in the lateral hip and hamstring. Hold for about 10 seconds. Repeat on the other side.

Supine Twist

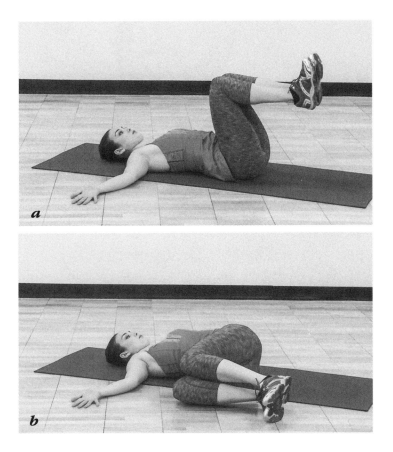

Lie on your back with your legs up and knees bent, shoulders on the floor, and arms out to the sides (see figure *a*). Drop your legs to one side while your shoulders remain on the floor and, if comfortable, turn your head to the right while relaxing your head and neck on the floor (see figure *b*). Take deep breaths and pull into the stretch a little deeper with each breath. Think about twisting from your center as you hold this stretch. Repeat on the other side.

Cat and Cow Stretch

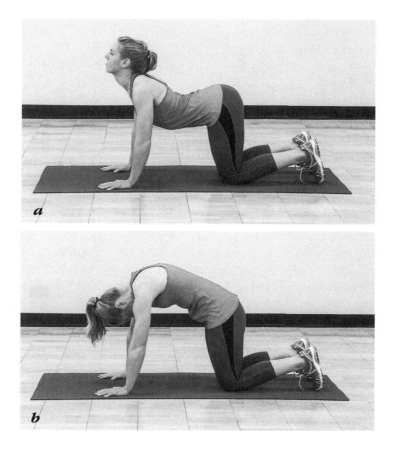

Place your hands directly under your shoulders with your knees hip-width apart. From this quadruped position, perform a cat stretch by arching your back and gently lifting your head to raise your chin while tucking your tailbone (see figure *a*). Hold the position for a few seconds, and then perform a cow stretch by tucking your chin and rounding out your back and exhaling (see figure *b*). Continue to move between these two postures for four to six repetitions.

REMEMBER YOUR TABATA GUIDELINES

As a quick recap, the Tabata HIIT guidelines are as follows:

- Max intervals include one exercise.
- Mixed intervals include the following:
  - If there are two exercises, perform exercise 1 for rounds 1 and 2, exercise 2 for rounds 3 and 4, exercise 1 for rounds 5 and 6, and exercise 2 for rounds 7 and 8.
  - If there are four exercises, perform exercise 1 for round 1, exercise 2 for round 2, exercise 3 for round 3, and exercise 4 for round 4; then repeat for rounds 5 through 8 in the same order.

HIIT WORKOUTS

The HIIT workouts in this section are broken down into 20-, 30-, and 45-minute workouts. You can choose based on how much time you have to exercise, your level of fitness, and your training goals. Many people consider longer workouts to be better workouts, but this is just not true, particularly with respect to HIIT. The fact that these workouts are short doesn't mean that they are any less effective than longer workouts. Short workouts are great to perform when you are pressed for time or are just starting out with HIIT. Additionally, because movement quality is the key to success, no matter which workouts you perform, if your movements are of high quality, your results will be fantastic.

These workouts are further divided into the HIIT protocols of max, mixed, and timing Tabata and the hard, harder, hardest formats. Following the timed workout sequences are 4-minute microburst Tabata workouts you can plug into any of your daily exercise routines. A great addition to any cardio workout, they are performed at the beginning (after a warm-up), in the middle, or at the end of a traditional steady-state routine. You can also perform them when you are pressed for time but still want to take advantage of the benefits of HIIT.

20-Minute Workouts

The five 20-minute body-weight workouts in this section are quick to perform and very effective; all are from the menus in chapter 8. One focuses on the lower body, one focuses on the lower body and core, two focus on the upper body and core, and one focuses on just the core.

Even though these routines focus on specific body parts, the entire body is involved in stabilization, strengthening, and burning calories. You will become breathless, crossing the anaerobic threshold, yet still be emphasizing a particular body part in these short but powerful workouts.

These workouts require nothing more than your own body weight, so make sure you have a clear area in which to exercise and, for the upper-body and core exercises, a mat for your knees and elbows for comfort if necessary. Also, be sure to have water available to drink anytime you feel thirsty, or to sip during your recovery between rounds or interval sequences.

20-Minute Workout 1
LOWER BODY

Use Tabata timing, and recover for 60 to 90 seconds between sequences.

▸ *Warm-up:* 3-5 minutes
▸ *Max interval 1:* Squat with elbow drive (pg. 48)—4 minutes
▸ *Mixed interval 1:* Basic squat (pg. 45); basic lunge (pg. 58)—4 minutes
▸ *Mixed interval 22:* Curtsy lunge (pg. 65); twist (pg. 76)—4 minutes
▸ *Cool-down/transition out:* 3 minutes

20-Minute Workout 2
LOWER BODY AND CORE

Use Tabata timing, and recover for 60 to 90 seconds between sequences.

▸ *Warm-up:* 3-5 minutes
▸ *Max interval 2:* Quarter-turn squat (pg. 51)—4 minutes
▸ *Mixed interval 7:* Squat jack (pg. 55); Brazilian lunge (pg. 62) —4 minutes
▸ *Mixed interval 24:* Bridge (pg. 133); full bicycle crunch (pg. 132) —4 minutes
▸ *Cool-down/transition out:* 3 minutes

20-Minute Workout 3
UPPER BODY AND CORE

Use Tabata timing, and recover for 60 to 90 seconds between sequences.

▸ *Warm-up:* 3-5 minutes
▸ *Max interval 3:* Two-knee push-up (pg. 91)—4 minutes
▸ *Mixed interval 9:* Wood chop squat (pg. 56); mountain climber (pg. 72)—4 minutes
▸ *Mixed interval 3:* Forearm plank (pg. 121); forearm side plank (pg. 122) —4 minutes
▸ *Cool-down/transition out:* 3 minutes

20-Minute Workout 4
UPPER BODY AND CORE

Use Tabata timing, and recover for 60 to 90 seconds between sequences.

- ▸ *Warm-up:* 3-5 minutes
- ▸ *Max interval 19:* Mountain climber (pg. 72)—4 minutes
- ▸ *Mixed interval 23:* Basic push-up (pg. 88); step-back burpee (pg. 126) —4 minutes
- ▸ *Mixed interval 6:* V-sit (pg. 127); full bicycle crunch (pg. 132)—4 minutes
- ▸ *Cool-down/transition out:* 3 minutes

20-Minute Workout 5
CORE

Use Tabata timing, and recover for 60 to 90 seconds between sequences.

- ▸ *Warm-up:* 3-5 minutes
- ▸ *Max interval 14:* Curtsy lunge (pg. 65)—4 minutes
- ▸ *Mixed interval 12:* Half bicycle crunch (left and right) (pg. 131); full bicycle crunch (pg. 132)—4 minutes
- ▸ *Mixed interval 9:* Wood chop squat (pg. 56); mountain climber (pg. 72) —4 minutes
- ▸ *Cool-down/transition out:* 3 minutes

30-Minute Workouts

These six 30-minute workouts include a variety of portable equipment options as well as body weight. These workouts are quick to perform and very effective; all are from the menus in chapter 8. Two of the workouts have a lower-body emphasis, two have an upper body and core emphasis, and two emphasize both the lower body and upper body. To balance the workouts, we have included at least one core sequence and one max interval in each.

Keep in mind that even though an exercise sequence may have a specific body part focus, you will still get a total-body workout, cross the anaerobic threshold, and need recovery between the interval sequences. Be prepared by having available all necessary equipment and a mat for your hands, arms, and knees, if necessary. Keep all equipment clear of your exercise area, and be sure to have water available to drink during your recovery sequences.

Note: When performing the hard, harder, hardest intervals, if the time is 2 minutes and 5 seconds, perform the interval sequence only once. If 4 minutes and 10 seconds are indicated, then perform the sequence twice, with a right and then a left lead.

30-Minute Workout 1
LOWER BODY

Use Tabata and hard, harder, hardest timing, and recover for 60 to 90 seconds between sequences.

- *Warm-up:* 3-5 minutes
- *Max interval 5:* Plié squat (pg. 53)—4 minutes
- *Hard, harder, hardest 1:* Basic squat (pg. 45); squat to heel raise (pg.46); squat jump (pg. 47)—2 minutes 5 seconds
- *Mixed interval 25:* Speedskater (pg. 74); squat jump (pg. 47)—4 minutes
- *Hard, harder, hardest 19:* Jumping jack with arms to front (pg. 78); mogul twist (pg. 75); speedskater (pg. 74)—2 minutes 5 seconds
- *Mixed interval 16:* Quarter-turn squat (pg. 51); messy lunge (pg. 63)—4 minutes
- *Mixed interval 30:* Wood chop (pg. 129); plank to pike (pg. 123)—4 minutes
- *Cool-down/transition out:* 3 minutes

30-Minute Workout 2
LOWER BODY

Use Tabata and hard, harder, hardest timing, and recover for 60 to 90 seconds between sequences.

- ▸ *Warm-up:* 3-5 minutes
- ▸ *Max interval 25:* Basic lunge (pg. 58)—4 minutes
- ▸ *Hard, harder, hardest 13:* Squat to heel raise (pg. 46); squat with elbow drive (pg. 48); plié squat (pg. 54)—2 minutes 5 seconds
- ▸ *Mixed interval 22:* Curtsy lunge (pg. 65); twist (pg. 76)—4 minutes
- ▸ *Mixed interval 7:* Squat jack (pg. 55); Brazilian lunge (pg. 62)—4 minutes
- ▸ *Hard, harder, hardest 28:* Front lunge with knee lift (pg. 68); messy lunge (pg. 63); twist (pg. 76)—2 minutes 5 seconds
- ▸ *Mixed interval 27:* V-sit with rotation (pg. 128); eagle wrap reverse crunch (pg. 130)—4 minutes
- ▸ *Cool-down/transition out:* 3 minutes

30-Minute Workout 3
UPPER BODY AND CORE

Use Tabata and hard, harder, hardest timing, and recover for 60 to 90 seconds between sequences.
Equipment: Tubing

- ▸ *Warm-up:* 3-5 minutes
- ▸ *Max interval 30:* Plank to pike (pg. 123)—4 minutes
- ▸ *Hard, harder, hardest 8:* Chest press (pg. 93); two-knee push-up (pg. 91); chest fly (pg. 95)—4 minutes 10 seconds
- ▸ *Mixed interval 14:* Seated row (pg. 100); single-arm biceps curl (pg. 108)—4 minutes
- ▸ *Mixed interval 11:* Chest press (pg. 93); lat pulldown (pg. 96)—4 minutes
- ▸ *Mixed interval 15:* Bridge (pg. 133); single-leg bridge (pg. 134)—4 minutes
- ▸ *Cool-down/transition out:* 3 minutes

30-Minute Workout 4
UPPER BODY AND CORE

Use Tabata and hard, harder, hardest timing, and recover for 60 to 90 seconds between sequences.
Equipment: Dumbbells, tubing

- ▸ *Warm-up:* 3-5 minutes
- ▸ *Max interval 24:* Jumping jack with arms to front (pg. 78)—4 minutes
- ▸ *Hard, harder, hardest 29:* Burpee with push-up (pg. 71); chest press (pg. 93); lat pulldown (pg. 96)—4 minutes 10 seconds
- ▸ *Mixed interval 18:* Plank (pg. 87); dolphin push-up (pg. 73)—4 minutes
- ▸ *Mixed interval 9:* Wood chop squat (pg. 56); mountain climber (pg. 72)—4 minutes
- ▸ *Hard, harder, hardest 17:* Biceps curl (pg. 107); single-arm biceps curl (pg. 108); lateral raise with dumbbells (pg. 105)—4 minutes 10 seconds
- ▸ *Cool-down/transition out:* 3 minutes

30-Minute Workout 5
LOWER AND UPPER BODY

Use Tabata and hard, harder, hardest timing, and recover for 60 to 90 seconds between sequences.
Equipment: Dumbbells, tubing

- ▸ *Warm-up:* 3-5 minutes
- ▸ *Max interval 12:* Brazilian lunge (pg. 62)—4 minutes
- ▸ *Hard, harder, hardest 5:* Basic push-up (pg. 88); chest press (pg. 93); triceps kickback (pg. 109)—4 minutes 10 seconds
- ▸ *Mixed interval 28:* Jumping jack with arms to front (pg. 78); mogul twist (pg. 75)—4 minutes
- ▸ *Mixed interval 26:* Single-arm bent-over row (pg. 99); upright row with dumbbells (pg. 103)—4 minutes
- ▸ *Mixed interval 24:* Bridge (pg. 133); full bicycle crunch (pg. 132)—4 minutes
- ▸ *Mixed interval 21:* Swimmer (pg. 125); plank with shoulder tap (pg. 120)—4 minutes
- ▸ *Cool-down/transition out:* 3 minutes

30-Minute Workout 6
LOWER AND UPPER BODY

Use Tabata and hard, harder, hardest timing, and recover for 60 to 90 seconds between sequences.

Equipment: Dumbbells

- ▸ *Warm-up:* 3-5 minutes
- ▸ *Max interval 10:* Cycle lunge (pg. 60)—4 minutes
- ▸ *Hard, harder, hardest 20:* Shoulder press (pg. 101); biceps curl (pg. 107); single-arm biceps curl (pg. 108)—4 minutes 10 seconds
- ▸ *Mixed interval 25:* Speedskater (pg. 74); squat jump (pg. 47)—4 minutes
- ▸ *Mixed interval 19:* Plié squat (pg. 53); single-leg balance lunge (pg. 64) —4 minutes
- ▸ *Max interval 7:* Wood chop squat (pg. 56)—4 minutes
- ▸ *Mixed interval 21:* Swimmer (pg. 125); plank with shoulder tap (pg. 120) —4 minutes
- ▸ *Cool-down/transition out:* 3 minutes

45-Minute Workouts

The five 45-minute workouts in this section include a variety of equipment and body-weight options. These workouts are quick to perform and very effective; all are from the menus in chapter 8. All five workouts emphasize the lower body, upper body, and core. Each workout includes at least one max interval and at least one core sequence. Because these workouts are longer, they vary in intensity more than the 20- and 30-minute workouts do.

Even though these workouts are longer than the previous ones, you will cross the anaerobic threshold and need recovery between the interval sequences. It is important to pace yourself, performing each round to the best of your ability and using the strategies for success described in earlier chapters.

Be prepared by having available the necessary equipment and a mat for your hands, arms, and knees, if necessary. Keep all equipment clear of your exercise area, and be sure to have water available to drink between interval sequences.

Note: When performing the hard, harder, hardest intervals, if the time is 2 minutes and 5 seconds, perform the sequence only once. If 4 minutes and 10 seconds are indicated, then perform the sequence twice, with a right and then a left lead.

45-Minute Workout 1
LOWER AND UPPER BODY

Use Tabata and hard, harder, hardest timing, and recover for 60 to 90 seconds between sequences.
Equipment: Dumbbells, tubing

- ▸ *Warm-up:* 3-5 minutes
- ▸ *Max interval 27:* Squat jump (pg. 47)—4 minutes
- ▸ *Hard, harder, hardest 7:* Brazilian lunge (pg. 62); messy lunge (pg. 63); front to back lunge (pg. 59)—4 minutes 10 seconds
- ▸ *Mixed interval 30:* Wood chop (pg. 129); plank to pike (pg. 123)—4 minutes
- ▸ *Hard, harder, hardest 10:* Squat jack (pg. 55); burpee, (pg. 57); plank with shoulder tap (pg. 120)—4 minutes 10 seconds
- ▸ *Hard, harder, hardest 14:* Military-style push-up (pg. 90); seated row (pg. 100); lateral raise with tubing (pg. 106)—4 minutes 10 seconds
- ▸ *Mixed interval 9:* Wood chop squat (pg. 56); mountain climber (pg. 72)—4 minutes
- ▸ *Hard, harder, hardest 26:* Single-arm bent-over row (pg. 99); upright row with dumbbells (pg. 103); single-arm biceps curl (pg. 108)—4 minutes 10 seconds
- ▸ *Cool-down/transition out:* 3-5 minutes

45-Minute Workout 2
LOWER AND UPPER BODY

Use Tabata and hard, harder, hardest timing, and recover for 60 to 90 seconds between sequences.

Equipment: Tubing

- ▸ *Warm-up:* 3-5 minutes
- ▸ *Max interval 21:* Mogul twist (pg. 75)—4 minutes
- ▸ *Hard, harder, hardest 25:* Burpee with vertical jump (pg. 70); basic lunge (pg. 58); single-leg balance lunge (pg. 64)—4 minutes 10 seconds
- ▸ *Hard, harder, hardest 16:* Diagonal lunge with floor touch (pg. 61); curtsy lunge (pg. 65); twist (pg. 76)—2 minutes 5 seconds
- ▸ *Mixed interval 14:* Seated row (pg. 100); single-arm biceps curl (pg. 108) —4 minutes
- ▸ *Hard, harder, hardest 8:* Chest press (pg. 93); two-knee push-up (pg. 96); chest fly (pg. 95)—4 minutes 10 seconds
- ▸ *Max interval 22:* Twist (pg. 76)—4 minutes
- ▸ *Mixed interval 10:* Side-to-side squat (pg. 52); squat to heel raise (pg. 46) —4 minutes
- ▸ *Mixed interval 12:* Half bicycle crunch (left and right) (pg. 131); full bicycle crunch (pg. 132)—4 minutes
- ▸ *Cool-down/transition out:* 3-5 minutes

45-Minute Workout 3
LOWER BODY AND CORE

Use Tabata and hard, harder, hardest timing, and recover for 60 to 90 seconds between sequences.

- ▸ *Warm-up:* 3-5 minutes
- ▸ *Max interval 6:* Squat jack (pg. 55)—4 minutes
- ▸ *Mixed interval 9:* Wood chop squat (pg. 56); mountain climber (pg. 72) —4 minutes
- ▸ *Hard, harder, hardest 12:* Plank to pike (pg. 123); half bicycle crunch (left and right) (pg. 131)—4 minutes 10 seconds
- ▸ *Max interval 23:* Power speed skip (pg. 77)—4 minutes
- ▸ *Mixed interval 25:* Speedskater (pg. 74); squat jump (pg. 47)—4 minutes
- ▸ *Mixed interval 22:* Curtsy lunge (pg. 65); twist (pg. 76)—4 minutes
- ▸ *Mixed interval 21:* Swimmer (pg. 125); plank with shoulder tap (pg. 120) —4 minutes
- ▸ *Hard, harder, hardest 27:* Mountain climber (pg. 72); plank (pg. 87); forearm side plank with reach (pg. 124)—4 minutes 10 seconds
- ▸ *Cool-down/transition out:* 3-5 minutes

45-Minute Workout 4
UPPER BODY AND CORE

Use Tabata and hard, harder, hardest timing, and recover for 60 to 90 seconds between sequences.
Equipment: Dumbbells, tubing

- *Warm-up:* 3-5 minutes
- *Max interval 3:* Two-knee push-up (pg. 91)—4 minutes
- *Max interval 22:* Twist (pg. 76)—4 minutes
- *Mixed interval 15:* Bridge (pg. 133); single-leg bridge (pg. 134)—4 minutes
- *Hard, harder, hardest 23:* Chest press (pg. 93); triceps push-up (pg. 89); plank (pg. 87)—2 minutes 5 seconds
- *Hard, harder, hardest 3:* V-sit (pg. 127); V-sit with rotation (pg. 128); full bicycle crunch (pg. 132)—2 minutes 5 seconds
- *Mixed interval 26:* Single-arm bent-over row (pg. 99); upright row with dumbbells (pg. 103)—4 minutes
- *Max interval 24:* Jumping jack with arms to front (pg. 78)—4 minutes
- *Hard, harder, hardest 23:* Chest press (pg. 93); triceps push-up (pg. 89); plank (pg. 87)—2 minutes 5 seconds
- *Hard, harder, hardest 11:* Lat pulldown (pg. 96); single-arm pulldown (pg. 97); upright row with tubing (pg. 104)—4 minutes 10 seconds
- *Cool-down/transition out:* 3-5 minutes

45-Minute Workout 5
LOWER AND UPPER BODY

Use Tabata and hard, harder, hardest timing, and recover for 60 to 90 seconds between sequences.
Equipment: Tubing, dumbbell

- *Warm-up:* 3-5 minutes
- *Max interval 16:* Front lunge with knee lift (pg. 68)—4 minutes
- *Max interval 28:* Burpee with vertical jump (pg. 70)—4 minutes
- *Hard, harder, hardest 22:* Cycle lunge (pg. 60); basic squat (pg. 45); plié squat with heel click (pg. 54)—2 minutes 5 seconds
- *Hard, harder, hardest 18:* Half bicycle crunch (left and right) (pg. 131); full bicycle crunch (pg. 132)—4 minutes 10 seconds
- *Hard, harder, hardest 4:* Lateral lunge with touch (pg. 66); lateral lunge with adduction (pg. 67); pendulum lunge (pg. 69)—2 minutes 5 seconds
- *Hard, harder, hardest 9:* Swimmer (pg. 125); bridge (pg. 133); single-leg bridge (pg. 134)—4 minutes
- *Mixed interval 5:* Bent-over row (pg. 98); biceps curl (pg. 107)—4 minutes
- *Mixed interval 17:* Push press (pg. 102); quadruped triceps press (pg. 110)—4 minutes
- *Cool-down/transition out:* 3-5 minutes

FOUR-MINUTE MICROBURST TABATA WORKOUTS

If you are hard-pressed for time, any of the following Tabata max intervals will create a quick high-intensity workout. These powerful 4-minute microburst intervals will do the trick when it comes to maintaining a high level of fitness through HIIT training. Don't underestimate their power; you need only perform one 4-minute interval sequence to get the benefits of high-intensity interval training. They aren't a substitution for full workouts, but they can be used once daily, or on days when you can't fit in a full HIIT workout. They can also be used as an adjunct to long runs, walks, and strength or yoga workouts.

Before performing any of these workouts, warm up for at least 1 minute. Remember, a max interval incorporates only one exercise, which you perform at your greatest effort for 20 seconds followed by 10 seconds of active or passive recovery before going again and again. Eight rounds constitute a full 4-minute max interval Tabata workout. Be sure to cool down and transition out before either moving on with your day or continuing to your next activity.

Squat with elbow drive (pg. 48)

Quarter-turn squat (pg. 51)

Two-knee push-up (pg. 91)

Side-to-side squat (pg. 52)

Plié squat (pg. 54)

Squat jack (pg. 55)

Wood chop squat (pg. 56)

Burpee (pg. 57)

Front to back lunge (pg. 59)

Cycle lunge (pg. 60)

Diagonal lunge with floor touch (pg. 61)

Brazilian lunge (pg. 62)

Messy lunge (pg. 63)

Curtsy lunge (pg. 65)

Lateral lunge with adduction (pg. 67)

Front lunge with knee lift (pg. 68)

Pendulum lunge (pg. 69)

Dolphin push-up (pg. 73)

Mountain climber (pg. 72)

Single-leg squat (pg. 50)

Mogul twist (pg. 75)

Twist (pg. 76)

Power speed skip (pg. 77)

Jumping jack with arms to front (pg. 78)

Basic lunge (pg. 58)

Plié squat with heel click (pg. 54)

Squat jump (pg. 47)

Burpee with vertical jump (pg. 70)

Speedskater (pg. 74)

Plank to pike (pg. 123)

CREATE YOUR OWN WORKOUTS

Creating your own workouts using the max interval, mixed interval, and hard, harder, hardest options in chapter 8 is very easy. Simply mix and match the exercises based on your preferences and exercise goals. Use the following template to put together the exercises any way you chose. This template is designed for a 20- to 30-minute workout; simply add or subtract exercises to create a time frame that fits your schedule. Don't forget to warm up before you start and cool down when you are finished.

Figure 10.1 Workout Creation Template

Warm-up	Interval 1	Interval 2	Interval 3	Interval 4
Lower-body focus				
Upper-body focus				
Core Focus				
Cool-down				

From I. Lewis-McCormick, The HIIT Advantage. (Champaign, IL: Human Kinetics).

NOT ENOUGH TIME?

The problem that many well-intentioned exercisers run into is that they don't have enough time to fit consistent workouts into their daily or weekly schedules. No matter what shape you are in now, or what you wish to train for, HIIT protocols are a time-efficient option because 20 to 45 minutes of exercise can be performed on one to three nonconsecutive days per week with amazing results. This is one reason HIIT protocols are so popular; you don't need significant amounts of time to get the benefits of exercise using these routines. And if you have even less time, just one 4-minute Tabata interval sequence a day will be enough to help you stay on track with your weight loss goals, and it will help improve your overall fitness. All of the routines in this book include cardiorespiratory and strength training components to offer you all the benefits of HIIT.

The success of a new fitness program depends on the foundation that you build it on. These HIIT workouts are designed to meet the ultimate goal of enhanced fitness and better health. If the 30- or 45-minute workouts are too much for you, begin with the 20-minute workouts, once or twice a week. If that is still too much, begin with one 4-minute Tabata interval each time you work out (3 to 5 days per week). This will help you establish an anaerobic fitness base from which you can progress to meet your fitness goals.

Remember that better is always better, so pay attention to movement quality over quantity and move only at a pace you can control. Use this information as a starting point, and take the initiative to learn more about the many types of exercise you can incorporate into your HIIT workouts.

REFERENCES

Coe, S. 2013. *Running my life*. London: Hodder & Stoughton.

Gibala, M. 2009. Molecular responses to high-intensity interval exercise. *Applied Physiology, Nutrition, and Metabolism* 34(3), 428-432.

Gibala, M.J., J.P. Little, M.J. MacDonald, and J.A. Hawley. 2012. Physiological adaptations to low-volume, high-intensity interval training in health and disease. *Journal of Physiology* 590 (5): 1077-1084.

Haltom, R.W., et al. 1999. Circuit weight training and its effects on excess postexercise oxygen consumption. *Medicine & Science in Sports & Exercise* 31, 1613-8.

Helgerud, J, K. Høydal, E. Wang, T. Karlsen, P. Berg, M. Bjerkaas, T. Simonsen, C. Helgesen, N. Hjorth, R. Bach, and J. Hoff. 2007. Aerobic high-intensity intervals improve V̇O₂max more than moderate training. *Medicine & Science in Sports & Exercise* 39(4):665-71.

Hill, A.V. 1931. Adventures in biophysics. Philadelphia: University of Pennsylvania Press.

Hill, A.V., and H. Lupton. 1923. Muscular exercise, lactic acid, and the supply and utilization of oxygen. *Quarterly Journal of Medicine* 16, 135.

Kravitz, L. 2014. Metabolic effects of HIIT. *IDEA Fitness Journal* 11(5), 16-18.

Mylrea, M. 2011. *Tabata bootcamp certification training manual*. Carlsbad, CA: Savvier Fitness.

Osterberg, K.L., and C.L. Melby. 2000. Effect of acute resistance exercise on postexercise oxygen consumption and resting metabolic rate in young women. *International Journal of Sport Nutrition and Exercise Metabolism* 10 (1), 71-81.

Perry, C.G., G.J. Heigenhauser, A. Bonen, and L.L. Spriet. 2008. High-intensity aerobic interval training increases fat and carbohydrate metabolic capacities in human skeletal muscle. *Applied Physiology, Nutrition, and Metabolism* 33(6):1112-23.

Reynolds, J.M., and L. Kravitz. 2001. Resistance training and EPOC. *IDEA Personal Trainer* 12(5), 17-19.

Schuenke, M.D., R.P. Mikat, and J.M. McBride. 2002. Effect of an acute period of resistance exercise on excess post-exercise oxygen consumption: Implications for body mass management. *European Journal of Applied Physiology* 86(5):411-7.

Slørdahl, S.A., V.O. Madslien, A. Støylen, A. Kjos, J. Helgerud, and U. Wisløff. 2004. Atrioventricular plane displacement in untrained and trained females. *Medicine & Science in Sports & Exercise* 36: 1871-1875.

Tabata, I., K. Nishimura, M. Kouzaki, Y. Hirai, F. Ogita, M. Miyachi, and K. Yamamoto. 1996. Effects of moderate-intensity endurance and high-intensity intermittent training on anaerobic capacity and V̇O₂max. *Medicine & Science in Sports & Exercise* 28(10):1327-30.

INDEX

T

Tabata, Izumi 29-30
Tabata timers 148
    four-minute microburst workouts 174
Tabata training. *See also* HIIT
    about 29-30
    and negative recovery 6
    four-minute workouts 174
    hard, harder, hardest protocol 32-33,
      141*f*
    history of 4
    in-workout recovery time 18
    max interval 30, 32t, 137-139
    mixed interval 31-32, 32t, 140*f*
    progressive and regressive options
      139
    recovery ratio for 15
    timing interval 32, 32*t*
    timing your sequences 148-149
tools and toys
    dumbbells 37
    gliding disks 37
    kettlebells 37
    medicine balls 36
    mini-trampolines 37
    music 148-149
    options and selection 149
    resistance tubing 36
    rollers 18-24

    safety guidelines for 35-36
    stability balls 36
    stopwatch or clock 148
    suspension trainer 36-37
    Tabata timers 148
training
    signs of overtraining 16
trampolines 37
transverse abdominis muscle (TVA) 115
trapezius muscle 82
triceps kickback 109
triceps push-up 89
twist, supine 162
twist exercise 76
two-knee push-up 91

U

upper body foundational movements. *See*
    exercises, upper-body
upright row with dumbbells 103
upright row with tubing 104

V

variety in core training 115
V-sit exercise 127
V-sit with rotation exercise 128

W

warming up 17*t*

warm-up guidelines 17*t*
wood chop exercise 129
wood chop squat 56
workouts. *See also* exercises; exercises,
    warm ups; workouts, cool down
    and transition out
    active recovery 151
    cool down and transition out 159-
      163
    creation template 175*f*
    exercise order 147
    four-minute Tabata workout 174
    increasing or decreasing impact 147
    lead leg changes 147-148
    20-minute HIIT workouts 164-166
    30-minute HIIT workouts 167-170
    45-minute HIIT workouts 171-173
    on-ramps and off-ramps 145-146
    recovery between intervals 148
    staying on task 148
    timing your sequences 148-149
    warming up 17*t*, 152-158
    workout creation template 175
workouts, cool down and transition out
    back-lying knee to chest 160
    cat and cow stretch 163
    straight-leg raise 160
    supine figure four 161
    supine twist 162

ABOUT THE AUTHOR

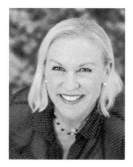

Irene Lewis-McCormick, **MS,** is a personal trainer, international presenter, author, and 30-year fitness veteran. She holds a master of science degree in exercise and sport science with an emphasis in physiology from Iowa State University. She is a certified strength and conditioning specialist with the National Strength and Conditioning Association and holds professional certifications from the Aerobics and Fitness Association of America, American College of Sports Medicine, American Council on Exercise, Aquatic Exercise Association, TRX, YogaFit, and many other organizations. Lewis-McCormick is the author of *A Woman's Guide to Muscle & Strength* (Human Kinetics, 2012) and faculty for SCW Fitness, ACSM, IDEA Health & Fitness, the Mayo Clinic, and many other international venues. She is a TRX suspension training master course trainer, a Tabata Bootcamp master trainer, an instructor for Barre Above and Xercise Lab, and a master instructor for JumpSport Fitness. She has been a featured presenter in several DVDs, including programs for pre- and postnatal exercise, water fitness, strength training,small-group training, circuit training, Pilates, and foam roller exercise. Lewis-McCormick is a contributor to consumer and fitness publications, including *Shape, More, IDEA Health & Fitness Journal, Prevention, Fitness Management, Diabetic Living, Diet,* and *Heart Healthy Living*. She is on the editorial advisory board of *Diabetic Living* magazine and is a subject matter expert and exam writer for the American Council on Exercise.

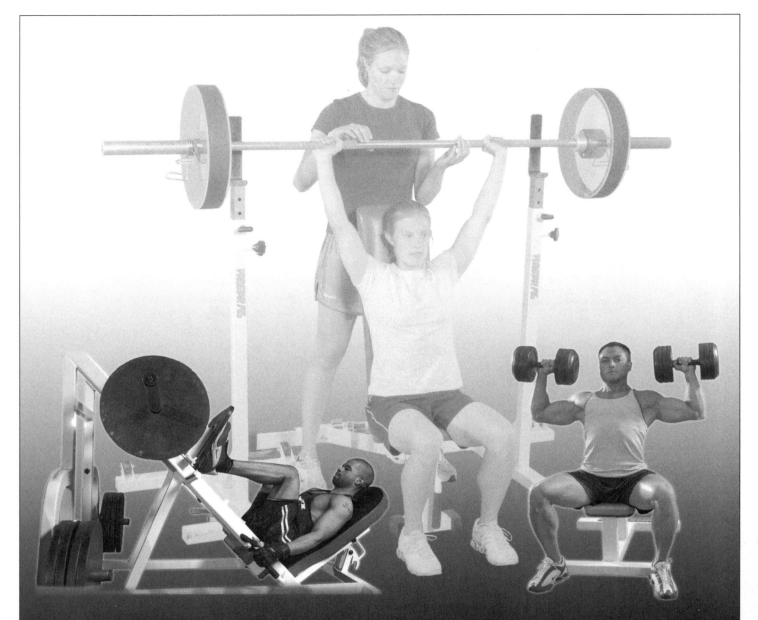

You'll find other outstanding strength training resources at

www.HumanKinetics.com/strengthtraining

In the U.S. call 1-800-747-4457

Australia 08 8372 0999 • Canada 1-800-465-7301
Europe +44 (0) 113 255 5665 • New Zealand 0800 222 062

 HUMAN KINETICS
The Premier Publisher for Sports & Fitness
P.O. Box 5076 • Champaign, IL 61825-5076 USA